MW00344727

THE
# ULTIMATE GUIDE
## TO PREVENTING AND TREATING
# MMA
# INJURIES

**FEATURING ADVICE FROM
UFC HALL OF FAMERS
RANDY COUTURE,
KEN SHAMROCK,
BAS RUTTEN,
PAT MILETICH,
DAN SEVERN
AND MORE!**

**JONATHAN GELBER, M.D., M.S.**

At ECW Press, we want you to enjoy this book in whatever format you like, whenever you like. Leave your print book at home and take the eBook to go! Purchase the print edition and receive the eBook free. Just send an email to ebook@ecwpress.com and include:

- the book title
- the name of the store where you purchased it
- your receipt number
- your preference of file type: PDF or ePub?

A real person will respond to your email with your eBook attached. And thanks for supporting an independently owned Canadian publisher with your purchase!

**Get the eBook free!***
*proof of purchase required

Copyright © Jonathan Gelber, 2016

Published by ECW Press
665 Gerrard Street East
Toronto, Ontario, Canada M4M 1Y2
416-694-3348 / info@ecwpress.com

All rights reserved. No part of this publication may be reproduced, stored in a retrieval system, or transmitted in any form by any process — electronic, mechanical, photocopying, recording, or otherwise — without the prior written permission of the copyright owners and ECW Press. The scanning, uploading, and distribution of this book via the Internet or via any other means without the permission of the publisher is illegal and punishable by law. Please purchase only authorized electronic editions, and do not participate in or encourage electronic piracy of copyrighted materials. Your support of the author's rights is appreciated.

This book is not intended as a substitute for the medical advice of a physician. The reader should regularly consult a physician in matters relating to his/her health and particularly with respect to any symptoms that may require diagnosis or medical attention. Please consult a physician before beginning any exercise regimen.

Editor for the press: Michael Holmes
Cover design: Michel Vrana
Cover image: Nicholas Piccolo/Shutterstock
Author photo: Michael Carotta
Interior exercise photos: Ryan Heckert/HexLinc Photos

LIBRARY AND ARCHIVES CANADA
CATALOGUING IN PUBLICATION

Gelber, Jonathan, author
The ultimate guide to preventing and treating MMA injuries : featuring advice from UFC Hall of Famers Randy Couture, Ken Shamrock, Bas Rutten, Pat Miletich, Dan Severn and more! / Jonathan Gelber, M.D., M.S.

Includes bibliographical references and index.
Issued in print and electronic formats.
ISBN 978-1-77041-172-2
also issued as: 978-1-77090-833-8 (pdf);
978-1-77090-834-5 (epub)

1. Martial arts injuries—Prevention.
2. Martial arts injuries—Treatment.

1. Title.

RC1220.M36G44 2016    617.1'02768    C2015-907270-0
C2015-907271-9

PRINTING: FRIESENS    5   4   3   2   1
PRINTED AND BOUND IN CANADA

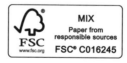

TO MY WIFE, CHILDREN, AND PARENTS
FOR THEIR LOVE AND SUPPORT.
AND TO THE ATHLETES AND COACHES
WHO SACRIFICE FOR THE SPORT.

CONTRIBUTORS/INTERVIEWEES (15 UFC TITLEHOLDERS, 6 UFC HALL
OF FAMERS, 32 MMA FIGHTERS, 7 ELITE TRAINERS, AND MORE)

Ken Shamrock (UFC HoF)

Frank Shamrock

Bas Rutten (UFC HoF)

Randy Couture (UFC HoF)

Sean Sherk

Dan Severn (UFC HoF)

Pat Miletich (UFC HoF)

Mark Coleman (UFC HoF)

Demetrious Johnson

Josh Barnett

Matt Serra

Carlos Condit

Carlos Newton

Tim Sylvia

Mark Hunt

Don Frye

Renzo Gracie

Gilbert Melendez

Matt Brown

Mario Sperry

Brandon Vera

Tim Kennedy

Dean Lister

Duane Ludwig

Jeff Monson

Pete Spratt

Stipe Miocic

Ed Herman

Nate Quarry

Guy Mezger

Patrick Côté

Matt Lindland

Stitch — MMA and boxing's
legendary cutman

Ricardo Liborio — Elite trainer/
coach, co-founder American Top
Team (ATT)

Cesar Gracie — Elite trainer/coach,
Cesar Gracie team

Mark DellaGrotte — Elite trainer/
coach, Team Sityodtong

Mike Winkeljohn — Elite trainer/
coach, Jackson-Winkeljohn team

Javier Mendez — Elite trainer/coach,
American Kickboxing Academy,
(AKA)

Greg Nelson — Elite trainer/coach,
the Academy

Ray Longo — Elite trainer/coach,
Serra/Longo competition team

"Big John" McCarthy — Referee and
advocate

Bruce Buffer — "The Voice of the
Octagon"

Andy Foster — Former fighter and
California Athletic Commissioner

FOREWORD BY A RINGSIDE DOC PIONEER
DR. JOE ESTWANIK // 1

INTRODUCTION AND BACKGROUND // 5

1.   HEAD TRAUMA AND PROLONGING YOUR CAREER // 9
   • NECK STRENGTHENING EXERCISES WITH STIPE MIOCIC // 24

2.   LACERATIONS AND THE CUTMAN'S BEST FRIEND // 27

3.   EYE INJURIES AND ORBITAL FRACTURES // 37
• THE FIGHTER'S CORNER: MENTAL PREPARATION BY FRANK SHAMROCK // 43

4.   KNEE INJURIES AND RETURNING TO THE OCTAGON AFTER SURGERY // 47
   • KNEE INJURY PREVENTION EXERCISES // 71

5.   SHOULDER INJURIES
AND HOW AN INJECTION CHANGED THE ODDS IN VEGAS // 79
   • SHOULDER INJURY PREVENTION EXERCISES // 94

6.   HIP INJURIES AND "THE HAMMER'S" HIP // 101
   • HIP STRENGTH AND FLEXIBILITY EXERCISES // 108
   • THE FIGHTER'S CORNER: A CAUTIONARY TALE BY KARO PARISYAN // 113

7.   HAND INJURIES AND MAKING APPLESAUCE BARE-HANDED // 117
   • THE FIGHTER'S CORNER: HAND WRAPPING
   WITH MARK DELLAGROTTE // 130

8.   SKIN INFECTIONS AND HOW MARK DELLAGROTTE SAVED *TUF* // 145

9.   WEIGHT-CUTTING, PEDS, AND TRT // 151

10.  INJURY PREVENTION: THE KEY LESSONS // 157
   • THE FIGHTER'S CORNER: STRUCTURING A TRAINING CAMP
   WITH GREG NELSON, DEMETRIOUS JOHNSON,
   AND PAT MILETICH // 180

INDEX // 183

# FOREWORD BY A RINGSIDE DOC PIONEER
## DR. JOE ESTWANIK, FORMER PRESIDENT AND CO-FOUNDER, ASSOCIATION OF RINGSIDE PHYSICIANS

As a young sports medicine doctor in the early 1980s, I was requested to assist as a ringside physician in a USA Boxing National Championship in my hometown. With my martial arts and wrestling background, I easily bonded with the athletes, coaches, officials, and refs. However, despite my enjoyment of the event, I felt something was off. The sports science available for this elite tournament was out of sync with what was then the current standard of sports medicine. I realized I needed to rapidly apply what we already knew in sports medicine to the boxing world. As I began to work on bringing science and medicine to the sport and to these athletes, I looked to my mentor Necip Apri, M.D. — a wizard at the fight game. It was amazing how often he could accurately predict outcomes and injuries! Soon, true ringside medicine was born, and I was at the forefront.

My interest allowed me to serve as chairman of sports medicine for USA Boxing and travel the world with our team for many years, including to Russia at the height of the Cold War. Then, suddenly out of Brazil came an "everything goes" combat — the early years of mixed martial arts. I quickly latched on to this great sport and was a ringside physician at *UFC 3* in 1994. Soon after, I worked as a team with the Gracie family, Big John McCarthy, and others to form MMA as we know it today. I helped establish rounds, referees, weight classes, and the number of fights per day for a competitor. I designed the original grappling glove with the help of my friends, particularly Big John McCarthy and John Perretti.

In the world of medicine, there is a "standard of care" that is applied to all athletes. These gold standards for injury prevention, recognition, and recovery are almost universally applied, irrespective of the sport. The knowledge currently available must be extended to and applied to athletes within traditional team sports, such as baseball, basketball, and football, as well as non-traditional and combat sports. A torn ACL in the knee of a football player is not different than a torn ACL in a wrestler's knee. A concussive impact from heading a soccer ball affects the same type of neurons disrupted from a punch that connects with a boxer's head. The many systemic disruptions created by starvation, dehydration, and incomplete rehydration affect all athletes, including wrestlers, boxers, MMA fighters, or even military warriors.

However, one must also keep in mind that each sport generates injuries and mechanisms of injury specific to the training and competition of the respective athletes. For example, the chapter on shoulder injuries excellently details exposure to pressures on the shoulder joint commonly produced by martial arts/boxing demands that may not be found in other sports. MMA athletes deserve a sports medicine team familiar with the specific demands, rules, mechanisms of injury, and rehabilitation techniques unique to the combat arts. The team should include coaches, certified athletic trainers, strength/conditioning coaches, nutritionists, and physicians familiar with the sport of MMA. My advice is to search out a doctor familiar with the demands of your sport. At the time of writing this, the Association of Ringside Physicians in conjunction with the American College of Sports Medicine have created a certification in ringside medicine that may be one guide to help you find a doctor familiar with boxing/

MMA. And always be wary of the doctor who would rather be your friend at an event than a doctor treating you as a patient.

As athletes, your responsibilities and duties span three time zones: pre-event, intra-event, and post-competition.

## PRE-EVENT

Choose your correct certified weight class by measuring your body fat percentage using skin calipers or other measures of hydration. Wrestling coaches and athletic trainers have measured many tens of thousands of competitors and are familiar with the tools available. Be judicious in the amount and aggressiveness of sparring. Training harder does not mean sparring harder. It is known that many of Muhammad Ali's detrimental impacts occurred during his vicious sparring sessions. Just as football coaches are recently limiting full-contact sessions, fighters should follow the same advice. Be honest to your coaches in declaring injuries, headaches, and concussions.

## INTRA-EVENT

Just as the referee serves as a neutral judge of the rules, the ringside physician referees your immediate and long-term health and safety. Listen to the referee or fight doctor if he stops a fight and accept his decision. It's better to live to fight another day!

## POST-COMPETITION

Cooperate with the ringside doctor's instructions for follow-up care. Even sub-concussive (non-knockouts) require physical and mental rest. You should avoid celebrating with alcohol consumption for several days after a bout, as recent studies note impaired brain-cell healing with alcohol. Seek experts in injury rehabilitation, such as physical therapists who understand the specific demands of your sport.

This book by Jonathan D. Gelber, M.D., M.S., shares his interest and expertise in sports medicine to educate those involved in mixed martial arts. The dedicated athletes of this ancient art do not deserve ancient science. The sound advice provided by Dr. Gelber illustrates the "gold standards" that you so deserve.

Joseph J. Estwanik, M.D., FACSM
Author of *Sports Medicine for the Combat Arts*
President of the Association of Ringside Physicians 2011–2014

# INTRODUCTION AND BACKGROUND

I have been a fan of mixed martial arts since before the term MMA even existed. I was first exposed to the ground game of grappling via classes in shootfighting and Gracie Jiu-Jitsu. I recall passing around videotapes of Pride and the early UFCs among our jiu-jitsu class, because not everyone could get the shows on their TV. You could only watch the UFC on satellite TV or buy Pride videos at f.y.e. in the mall. I also searched eagerly for the legendary *Gracie in Action* videotapes showing the birth of Gracie Jiu-Jitsu in Brazil. Fast-forward 15 years, and MMA is one of the world's fastest growing sports with shows or bouts on TV almost any night of the week and major cards happening almost weekly.

As the sport evolved from the early wars of strictly Brazilian Jiu-Jitsu versus American wrestling (think Royce Gracie versus Dan Severn or Ken Shamrock) to the gradual inclusion of Muay Thai strikers, the training of fighters has also evolved. From the pioneers of mixed martial arts, whose main goal was to be the toughest or strongest guy in the gym, elite, versatile athletes have emerged, training year round in strength, conditioning, cardio, and technique in one of the most physically demanding sports on the planet. Unfortunately, while the fighters have evolved, the support system around them has not. When it comes to many areas of injury prevention and treatment, MMA is still stuck in the Dark Ages.

As a doctor, fan, and participant, I began to notice that there is not a lot of good advice out there for the MMA athlete. As a result, athletes merely ignore their injuries or take the advice of a well-meaning but self-proclaimed expert whom they train with at their gym — not always the best source of information. In my experience, many mixed martial artists do not have insurance or do not think traditional medical doctors have much to offer them — but nothing could be further from the truth. MMA fighters are very in touch with their bodies, and many prefer a holistic approach to their health, but ignoring science and medicine puts them at risk for a shorter career.

The medical community has learned a lot about injury prevention from mainstream sports such as baseball, football, basketball, and soccer. And because of that, these million-dollar athletes rely on their team's athletic trainers, physical therapists, and team doctors for advice. But the MMA community hasn't yet adequately applied this knowledge to our sport, and with even more cards and more fighters eager to get on pay-per-view or fight for a world title, the number of injuries in MMA is rising. Without the proper education on injury prevention and treatment, many fighters develop tunnel vision and focus only on the fight in front of them. They do not pay attention to their bodies and the long-term consequences of their actions and training routines. And when their careers abruptly end or their bodies begin to break down, they struggle to remain relevant in the MMA world. However, with the help of a trained support system, these fine athletes will be able to prolong their careers and limit the chronic injuries they will have to deal with when they retire.

In order to help educate fighters, fans, and trainers, I began my website FightMedicine.net. Through my interaction with readers, many of whom come from all levels of MMA organizations, I realized there weren't enough adequate resources for members of the MMA community to turn to for advice. Thus, I decided to use my medical training and passion for the sport to write a book on MMA injuries, treatment, and prevention. To do that, I interviewed many UFC titleholders and Hall of Famers, MMA legends, current fighters, and their trainers. The advice they provided coupled with sound medical information will benefit both the current and next generation of mixed martial artists. MMA athletes deserve the same level of sports medicine as athletes in more traditional sports. I, along with many other medical professionals and scientists, want to see this sport grow safely and the careers of these athletes last as long as possible.

Rather than create a laundry list of all the possible injuries that could occur in MMA, I have instead focused on some of the more common injuries based on what I have seen as a doctor, what appears in the news, and what has stood out among fighters. In addition, I have included some injuries I find interesting, some that can seriously affect a fighter's ability to return to the cage, and others that can be prevented with proper training.

In my many hours of interviews with current MMA fighters, retired legends, and some of the top trainers in the sport, a few themes repeatedly came up in the conversation. Sometimes, it was as if I had pressed play on a recorded interview from someone else. While the advice may seem obvious or simple on the surface, the actual application of these guidelines to MMA training is often overlooked or not deeply understood by the fighter and his team. Based on my research, the top five principles of injury prevention are:

1. Choose the right camp and surround yourself with good people.
2. Use proper equipment in all aspects of training.
3. Listen to your body (not your ego) and adapt.
4. Avoid overtraining.
5. Train smarter, not harder.

Jonathan D. Gelber, M.D., M.S.
founder of FightMedicine.net
and the MMA Research Society

## CHAPTER 1

# HEAD TRAUMA AND
# PROLONGING YOUR CAREER

## CONCUSSIONS

The face of a fighter often tells their biography. Broken noses and cauliflower ears are usually tell-tale signs of a career in combat sports. These common injuries, however, are often only superficial. Much of the damage of a career in a combat sport such as MMA is under the surface. Concussion and brain injury are serious issues and more attention needs to be paid to the symptoms fighters experience. Instead of seeking treatment after a concussion, fighters chalk it up to simple run-of-the-mill injury and try to go on with their usual routine, even when something feels off.

MMA legend and pioneer Frank Shamrock admits to misunderstanding the severity of brain injuries as he describes his fight against Yuki Kondo in 1996 at Pancrase in Japan: "After 12 exhausting minutes of non-stop fighting, Yuki kicked me in the face and knocked me backwards. I fell through the second rope and hit my head on the metal floor. It knocked me out for about two seconds and they called the fight. That's the only time I ever got knocked out. I got up and felt woozy. I was sick to my stomach. I recovered pretty quickly and went out that night and had a good time. The next morning, I woke up and starting walking out of my hotel room. When I went to grab the doorknob, I found it was two inches to the left of where I grabbed. All that day in Japan, it kept happening. I flew home the next day and it still kept happening."

Another unfortunate example of not recognizing the symptoms of a concussion occurred at *UFC 17*. At that event, Lion's Den fighter Pete Williams fought former UFC Heavyweight Champion Mark Coleman in the main event. Pete's perfectly placed kick was the first-ever head-kick KO in UFC and has become one of the top knockouts in UFC history. Not long after the knockout, it seemed as though Mark had recovered, and neither Mark nor his team recognized the symptoms of a concussion until later that night. "I remember getting knocked out by Pete Williams. I got hit right in the kisser, and I'll tell you, he knocked "The Hammer" down. I was out cold for what felt like a good two minutes or so, but I got back up and left the Octagon. Back in the locker room, I was talking to my family for at least an hour when I suddenly stopped and looked at my dad and asked him why Big John stopped the fight. Up until then, I couldn't remember. And then things suddenly became clear again. My brain snapped back on. I had been talking to everyone for an hour, and no one realized my brain wasn't working completely."

## ANATOMY

In recent years, a lot of media attention has been focused on concussions in all sports. The brain is a soft-tissue organ encased in a hard, bony skull. A direct impact to the head such as a kick, a punch, or even a fall backwards onto the canvas imparts energy into the brain and skull. When this happens, the skull can either move faster or slower than the brain. When the skull eventually stops moving, conservation of momentum causes the brain to continue to move towards the skull. With enough force, the brain can slam into the skull (called a "coup" injury). Sometimes the brain even bounces back and hits the opposite side of the skull as well (a "contrecoup" injury).

As the brain smashes up against the skull, small areas of nerve connection can tear or stretch. Injured cells also release stimulating chemical signals that excite other nerve cells. The result is a chaotic highway of altered brain signaling, in which some cells die and others perform poorly for extended periods of time. And while those cells attempt to heal, a second injury (termed "second-impact syndrome") can be all the more deadly. That's why an athlete who suffers a concussion must be removed from a game. And not all concussions are caused by a knockout. Taking a lot of punishment standing up or even being "out on your feet" can result in either a concussion or "sub-concussive" episode even if the fighter doesn't lose via an actual KO. Famed MMA and Muay Thai coach Mark DellaGrotte remarks that, "It's more than just the guy who gets knocked out that you need to worry about. Sometimes the worst punches aren't the ones that knock you out, because at least with a knockout it's definitive. A lot of damage that these guys suffer is often overlooked. At least with a knockout, you see something you need to address."

## AWARENESS IS VITAL TO YOUR CAREER

Awareness that concussions can occur with or without a knockout, especially in boxing or MMA, is something important to understand. Strikeforce champion Gilbert Melendez recalls his experience with concussion symptoms without ever getting knocked out. "I've been knocked out once in practice, by Jake Shields, about eight to 10 years ago. With that knockout, I didn't have any headache or symptoms. But then I had a fight where I never went out, but afterwards I had a concussion. My head hurt and I had nausea. The symptoms lasted one week. Now, I try to avoid heavy sparring. In my younger years, I sparred more. But now I don't need to bang so hard. The smart people with a good coach will limit their sparring. And I tell people that's why you need a coach. When you are your own head coach, it's hard to limit yourself."

Keeping watch for concussion symptoms needs to continue well after the fight is over. In his rubber match with Andrei Arlovski at *UFC 61*, Tim Sylvia defeated "The Pit Bull" via unanimous decision to retain his UFC Heavyweight Championship. Arlovski is known as a hard striker, and despite not getting knocked out during the battle, Tim felt the effects of a concussion that night. "I think I have had a couple concussions, but the worst one I had was against Arlovski. We went the distance, and I went to bed that night. In the middle of the night, I got up to use the bathroom and had a head-rush and passed out right on the bathroom floor. I came to, went to try to go to bed, but passed out again and fell face first right back on the floor. My girlfriend found me on the floor and called the paramedics. The ambulance rushed me to the hospital and the doctor told me I had a concussion. I had to follow no contact for six months."

After a knockout or a concussion, a fighter may feel disoriented or confused. This is part of a post-concussion syndrome of multiple symptoms that may take anywhere from only a few seconds to as long as weeks or months to resolve. The symptoms may even develop or get worse over time, which is why it is imperative to look out for these symptoms after any knockout, even in training. Because the symptoms may not be overtly noticeable right away, ringside physicians should make it a point to talk to the fighters before their bouts, so they have a baseline of how they normally speak to use as a comparison later on after the fight. Coaches and training partners can do the same. Famed UFC announcer and kickboxer Bruce Buffer describes his own experience with sparring too hard too often, resulting in slurred speech — which can be a real problem for the "Voice of the Octagon." "Concussions are a scary thing. When I went to my doctor at 32 with what I felt was my second concussion from heavy sparring, he immediately told me to stop as the symptoms of slurred speech I experienced would potentially become much worse and possibly permanent if I continued. Plus it probably was not my first concussion; so I stopped contact and just trained non-contact from that point on."

Recognition of a concussion requires vigilance and familiarity with symptoms. Below is a list of concussion symptoms that may appear right after a knockout and others that may take some time to develop and appear.

Symptoms that may appear promptly after injury:

- Confusion
- Amnesia
- Headache
- Dizziness
- Ringing in the ears
- Nausea or vomiting
- Slurred speech
- Fatigue

Symptoms that may appear later:

- Memory or concentration problems
- Sensitivity to light and noise
- Sleep disturbances
- Irritability
- Depression

MMA legend Renzo Gracie has experienced some of these symptoms, having been knocked out twice in his career, "once by Dan Henderson and once against Matt Hughes. When it happened, I didn't feel anything. The lights just went off. I didn't have headaches or amnesia. But I know guys who have had those. I know one fighter who fought and finished a fight and didn't even remember what happened afterwards. That's scary." Former UFC fighter, King of the Cage Middleweight Champion, and world-class grappler Dean Lister weighs in: "I have had several concussions in my life. Some were from American football and others were from getting hit in the head in boxing and MMA. They are a mysterious thing to me. Sometimes they hurt badly right away but even then you usually won't know the true effects until later. I have had times, even for a few weeks, where I felt off balance and felt like collapsing. This is not to be underrated at all and can be serious. In hindsight, now that we know more about concussions, I should have seen a doctor right away. If anyone has these symptoms, please be very careful and please do not subject yourself to more abuse involving the brain. Yes, this means no sparring in boxing or kickboxing until cleared by a doctor trained in concussions. Not being aware of these symptoms and not educating yourself can be more dangerous than almost anything in MMA."

You may think your brain is doing fine, or you may not notice the small changes in mood, concentration, or reaction time. Or maybe your significant other tells you that you are forgetting things more often. These are all signs of long-term brain injury, and we are just starting to understand the causes. There is currently no standard test such as a blood sample or lumbar tap to detect levels of brain injury. However, an MRI may pick up brain changes that you were not aware of that can and should be monitored for changes by a brain injury physician.

## INJURY PREVENTION

Renzo Gracie understands that knockouts are a part of the sport, but he believes a fighter is most at risk for head injury during training sessions. "When it comes to getting knocked out in training, don't be a tough guy who gets knocked out and then keeps training. In fact, I think it's the training time that is the most dangerous. You train every day for a fight, but the actual fight is only 35 minutes long. As a coach, I noticed that once a guy gets knocked out, he gets knocked out a lot easier after that. A lot of coaches think they need to push a fighter 100% of the time. A fighter doesn't need to be hit every day. I look at the Russians training only 75–80% and then go on to win. The coach has an obligation to look at a fighter and make sure their career is long. This includes limiting their head injuries."

### WEAR HEADGEAR

While head strikes are part of the game, unnecessary concussions are not. Prevention begins with wearing appropriate headgear while training under adequate supervision. Coach Mike Winkeljohn, head striking-coach for Greg Jackson's elite team of fighters, including UFC champions Jon Jones and Holly Holm, says that prevention of head trauma goes beyond just the fighter — it involves the whole team, coaches included. "Coaches need to communicate with the fighters and watch the fighters and their energy levels. If they are getting tired and aren't performing, they're done. They are not proving anything other than how tough they are, and it's not benefiting anyone, especially the fighter. One of the biggest mistakes fighters make while training is they spar hard too much. They try to do too much in one day, get tired, and then their hands drop down. When their hands drop down, they take more trauma to head."

## LIMIT SPARRING

In addition to wearing headgear, being smart about how often and when you spar can help prevent concussions and head injuries. As Winkeljohn recommends, "In our camp, we only spar hard one time a week. During our camps, we used to spar hard twice a week. Then we noticed more knockouts and knockdowns later in the week. When guys spar hard, it affects them all week, and all kinds of injuries can happen. I have also noticed that with too much hard sparring, their focus and reaction time goes down and guys get tired easily. You also have to be a responsible training partner. I am a big believer in full-speed training, but once you hurt someone, you need to let up. Fighters always want to fight, so it's the guys around them that need to help them focus on the long term. The people around them should be held accountable."

Jackson-Winkeljohn MMA fighter Carlos Condit has limited his sparring as he has grown as a fighter. "This is something I have been thinking a lot about the last four to five years. Growing up, I would spar as much as I could, most of the time without headgear. Fighters like to fight, and even if it's a sparring session, it turns into a fight. It's good to have that fire inside you, but you need to hold yourself back. The more wars you have in the gym, the shorter your career. At Jackson's MMA, we only spar hard, all out, once every one to two weeks. Instead, we do heavy-intensity grappling with lots of movement. If we do add strikes, we put on the smaller MMA gloves, so no one is swinging too hard."

## GOING LIVE AND GOING HARD

Josh Barnett has a long history in MMA, including victories in Pride and defeating Randy Couture at age 24 for the UFC Heavyweight Championship. During that time, he has developed a practical philosophy on balancing hard or live training with knockouts. "In this sport, you will get hurt. You will get knocked out and get a concussion. I stepped into this knowing that. But you can limit the damage you receive. You have to go live during training, but you can go 70% or you can do drills where you let one guy win, which helps technique and preparation for a full-on fight. Without contact, you can't find that level of relaxation where you can avoid injury when you are out there. Contact helps you deal with your opponent's aggression better and teaches you to [reduce the intensity of] a punch by slipping it or taking some of the power out of it by rolling with the punch. That can't happen without live training. If I am sparring, I think 'Do I need to hit this guy in the head as hard a possible?' Usually the answer is 'no.' I can hit them harder in the body, but when I hit the face and head, I hit 60–70%. Knocking out my partner doesn't help me train — and then I lose a training partner."

Andy Foster is a former professional mixed martial artist and the executive director of the California State Athletic Commission, California's MMA regulatory body. As a former fighter who now looks at things from a regulatory and safety standpoint, he knows that every knockdown or knockout needs to be properly addressed. "If you are knocked down from a strike you should take some time off from sparring. If you are actually 'knocked out,' stop training and consult your physician immediately before returning. Once, when I was just simply knocked down during training, I saw my doctor and couldn't actually return to training for three weeks."

## LOSING YOUR CHIN

Cesar Gracie, who has coached top fighters such as the Diaz brothers, Gilbert Melendez, and Jake Shields, warns against going out there and swinging for the fences all the time. Because once you get knocked out and "lose your chin," there is no coming back. You can go from a top guy or champion to a low-level guy quickly. "The fans love guys who get in there and bang, but you have to be careful with the head damage you take. If you are going to spar, you need to spar light. There are a lot of tough-guy sayings about getting used to having your bell rung, but you don't need to get used to getting hit hard in the head. When it comes to your brain, it doesn't get stronger from getting hit. It only can get hurt. I have always been a fan of the intelligent fighter. I am a fan of the sport, but I don't want people to get beat up by over-sparring. And once your chin goes, it's gone. There's nothing you can do about it. Now all of a sudden you get hit with punches you could take before and suddenly the lights start going off. You get knocked out by easier punches."

Founder of the successful MMA camp American Kickboxing Academy, Javier Mendez, takes knockdowns in training seriously. "We spar Monday, Wednesday, and Friday, and unless you have a fight coming up, or we need you for something specific, we keep you out of the hard contact room and in the technique room. Most of our fighters elect to go one or two of those days with the smaller gloves, which we use to promote lighter contact. As a coach or trainer, you have to watch out for knockdowns. In our camp, if a fighter gets knocked down, it's an automatic 30-day suspension from sparring in our gym unless you get cleared from a doctor. I would rather be safe than sorry and use physicians as our number one resource for injury advice."

## AVOID SPARRING WITH HEAVIER OPPONENTS

Another training condition that puts fighters at risk of injury, especially excessive head trauma, is having fighters of largely different weight classes spar. While it may be good practice and an ego booster to fight a larger opponent, being significantly outweighed can lead to unnecessary heavy blows. Don Frye, MMA veteran and winner of two UFC tournaments, including the *Ultimate Ultimate 1996* tournament, sees this as a common mistake trainers make. "I have seen trainers at gyms do some dangerous things. One of these is having guys spar with more than 25–50 pounds difference. When an athlete becomes tired or hurt and can't raise his arms to fully protect his head and chin, it puts him at risk, and it's amplified [when fighting] bigger guys. Granted I am old school, but even I know better than that!"

## BASELINE TESTING LIKE THE PROS

Fighters may also consider getting baseline neurocognitive testing, which is what athletes in the NFL and NCAA do. This allows doctors and trainers to assess where a fighter or other athlete is in their recovery from a concussion and whether they are back at their baseline. You may not notice the subtle symptoms that these tests look for. The pendulum of treatment for concussions has swung in a different direction than previous generations. For a long time, athletes with concussions were instructed to lie quietly in a dark room and be woken up in the middle of the night. Current research suggests that the brain does need rest, but complete isolation is detrimental to a recovering brain. Most concussion specialists work with an athlete to determine how and when their symptoms arise and slowly push the limits as they feel comfortable until they can return to full competition.

## PRACTICAL ADVICE FROM A VETERAN

UFC tournament champion and Pride veteran Guy Mezger has spent several years working with professionals on brain health. "I consult with the Carrick Brain Center in Dallas and I am seeing more and more contact athletes being treated there. MMA athletes generally take fewer blows to the head during a match than most other fighting athletes, but it's the training that is the real killer." Some of Mezger's ideas for maintaining a healthy brain for the MMA athlete include:

- Do not use sparring as your method of conditioning. Work on technique specifics while sparring, but stay fresh. Use other training methods for conditioning such as Thai pad work, focus mitt work, bag work, sprinting, or high-intensity intervals.
- Save the really hard contact fighting for the actual fight. Don't wear your brain (and body) out in the gym.
- Strengthen your neck. A strong neck can be a shock absorber for the head.
- Cut massively down on alcohol, all drugs, and late-night partying. Make a decision to either be a fighter or a partier. It will undoubtedly cost you in the long run if you try to be both.
- Be nutritionally sound. There are a lot of nutritional supplements and foods that are brain protective in nature.
- If you do get your bell rung, be sure to get checked out and take the adequate time off. You do not want to sustain an injury in training and carry that over into the fight itself, putting yourself at further risk.
- Get to know a good neurologist and get CT scans or MRIs if prescribed. Often times you don't know what's brewing under the surface.

Guy's last point is particularly important as we slowly begin to understand the long-term consequences of traumatic brain injury. You may think your brain is doing fine, or you may not notice the small changes in mood, concentration, or reaction time. Or maybe your significant other tells you that you are forgetting things more often. These are all signs of long-term brain injury, whose causes we are just starting to understand. There is currently no standard simple test such as a blood sample or lumbar tap to detect levels of brain injury. However, an MRI may pick up brain changes that you were not aware of that can and should be monitored for changes by a brain injury physician.

Advocates for fighter health realize concussions are a big issue those involved in the sport need to address, especially as the earlier generations retire. As they get older, the signs of long-term traumatic brain injury can become significant. Understanding the long-term effects of traumatic brain injury and how we can limit them is something that is an active area of research, but until we have developed a test to detect levels of brain injury, simply being aware that there are long-term consequences is a first step in the right direction. "Big John" McCarthy, one of the sport's top referees inside the Octagon, is also an advocate for fighter safety and rule formation outside the cage. "The single most impactful injury to a combat sport athlete is usually a concussion. Although the fan sees things differently, anyone who has been affected by a concussion, especially fighters who are now retired and willing to put their shield of invincibility down, will tell you about the adverse effects that head trauma can bring into their lives. A fan sees a fighter break a leg or an arm, or dislocate an elbow, and they become almost ill at the sight of the injury. But many of the injuries in MMA do not carry the long-lasting effect that a concussion can carry.

"The fan sees a fighter get knocked unconscious and they get concerned for the fighter, but as soon as the fighter stands up and begins walking around, everyone feels better about the situation because they think, 'The fighter's okay.' It's a nice thought, but the truth is, the fighter is far from okay. If a fighter breaks their arm, everyone understands why they are out of the gym for the next eight weeks while their injury heals, but if a fighter is knocked out, we have no problem seeing them back in the gym one week after their fight. This, simply put, is crazy. Often times, a fighter who has received a concussion should be taking as much, if not more, time off for their injury than the fighter who suffers a more visible injury. Significant head trauma is arguably the most serious injury a fighter can absorb in their career. It changes their career. It changes their abilities in and out of the cage, and sometimes, it changes them as a person for the rest of their lives."

Big John brings up an excellent point. Many fighters and trainers have expressed the importance of prolonging your career, but many fighters only think about their next fight and not their life once they retire. Repeated head injury can lead to forgetfulness and mood disorders. The media is full of stories of NFL players or other athletes who suffered concussions throughout their career and ended up in deep states of depression, which in some cases led to suicide. This is certainly a tragic issue and is being investigated from a scientific standpoint. Autopsies of many of these athletes have found signs of chronic brain damage that may have led to their changes in personality. This may be a result of frontal lobe dysfunction — a

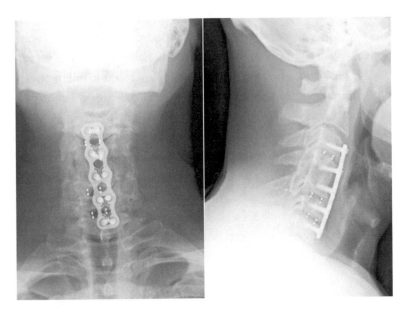

X-RAYS OF KEN SHAMROCK'S NECK SHOWING SURGICALLY FUSED CERVICAL VERTEBRAE. PHOTO COURTESY OF KEN SHAMROCK

reduction in the activity of the brain's front lobe, which usually limits our aggression and acts as a filter to our actions. We used to refer to chronic brain damage from combat sports as either dementia pugilistica, or punch-drunk syndrome, but now we refer to it as chronic traumatic encephalopathy, or CTE.

While we can begin to identify and recognize the clinical signs of CTE, it is only with an autopsy that we can definitively diagnose it. Scientists are looking into other ways to detect this type of brain damage, but until we have those tools available, athletes need to realize that long-term traumatic brain damage can lead to depression, forgetfulness, aggression, and other personality changes long after their MMA career is over. Sparring hard too much can make you lose your chin and can lead to shorter fights while inside the ring, but holding back during practice will undoubtedly help you lengthen your career and live a more fulfilled life outside the Octagon.

## KEEP YOUR NECK STRONG

Mike Winkeljohn says one of the most important things fighters can do to prevent knockouts and improve their ability to take a punch is to strengthen their neck muscles. But there is a fine line between strengthening the neck and putting yourself at risk for injury. "I have noticed the guys that do the best with neck exercises use slow, controlled movements." Retired MMA fighter Frank Shamrock agrees with keeping things light when dealing with the neck. "The best neck strengthening exercises are the ones that use only a little resistance."

When a fighter is hit in the head, significant forces are transmitted through the neck. Years of hard training and fighting can lead to deterioration of the cartilage and the cervical spine (discs in the neck), which can result in narrowing of the joint spaces, pain, and/or nerve impingement. Ken Shamrock is just one example of many fighters who have had to undergo surgical fusion of the cervical spine after years of pain.

Keeping your neck muscles strong may help prevent the traumatic forces a fighter's neck sees from wearing away the cartilage between the vertebrae. Ken credits his strong neck muscles with the longevity of his entire athletic career, not just MMA. "The only reason I was able to play football and become a pro fighter was because I made the areas of my injuries stronger so the muscle protected the site of my injury, including my neck muscles. Even after my career, I can't stop training because the areas of my body I have injured before become weak and then those same areas become more of a problem for me." Ken brings up a point that other chapters will explore, namely building up the muscles around a potentially injured area, not only to protect it, but to rehab an injury as well.

Pat Miletich has also had life-changing neck and spinal cord injuries from MMA. "While I was training to fight Frank Trigg, I got hit with a left hook. I immediately felt a crunch and the left side of my body went numb. I finished the round with my right hand. When I went to the doctor, an MRI showed my spinal canal was narrow, and it didn't leave a lot of room left for my spinal cord. I still have a lot of mobility but cannot take blunt force trauma to the forehead. I feel paralyzed when that happens. That's the reason I don't even spar anymore. It's not worth the risk of permanent injury. But I did learn some good exercises for strengthening my neck muscles. Sometimes I take my tongue and push it against roof of my mouth, which helps to activate the muscles. I use heavy bands for resisted movement, and I also push my head against a swiss exercise ball."

When doing neck exercises, a fighter should be careful of the more traditional exercises that have you putting your weight on the crown of your head. UFC legendary champion Randy Couture has some advice on this: "As far as your neck is concerned, avoid any and all exercises that put you on the crown of your head and compress the cervical spine. Long term, this puts stress on the cervical discs, which may cause them to degenerate, creating nerve and neck issues. Regular stretching can prevent and alleviate some of these issues."

# NECK STRENGTHENING EXERCISES

Strengthening your neck may help with brain injury prevention, but putting too much weight on your neck can lead to long-term damage. As Golden Glove winner and UFC Heavyweight Stipe Miocic demonstrates, you can use your own body to create resistance to make your neck muscles stronger.

Place your hand on the sides of your head, in front, or behind and push for resistance.

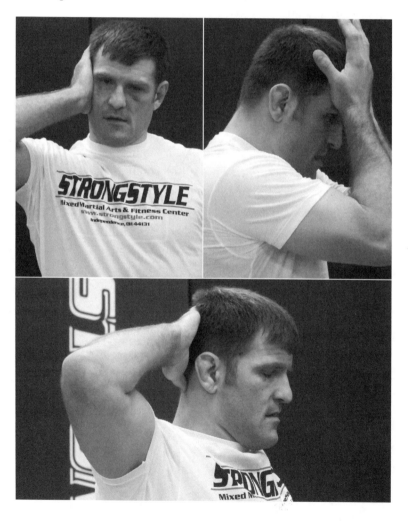

Lie on your side and lift your head sideways up against gravity.

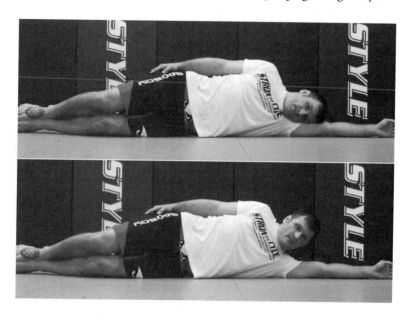

Push an exercise ball against a wall sideways or backwards.

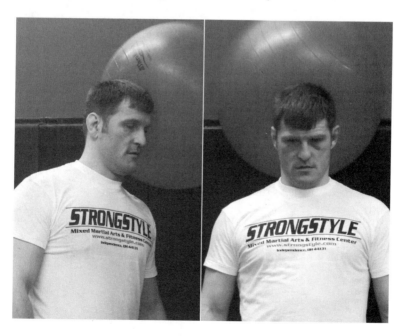

Push your head at an angle against the ball and rotate your head for rotational resistance. This also mimics strike avoidance.

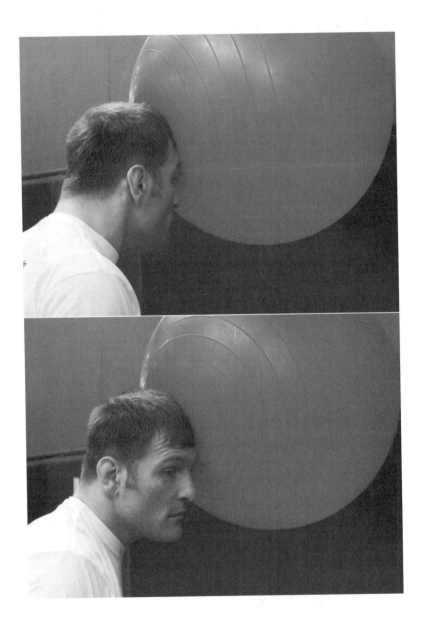

## CHAPTER 2

## LACERATIONS AND THE CUTMAN'S BEST FRIEND

### LACERATIONS – AKA "CUTS"

Veteran UFC trainer Mark DellaGrotte recounts his experience with his UFC fighter Marcus Davis and his bouts with recurrent lacerations: "Marcus Davis's problem is his buildup of scar tissue. He was always getting cut in training and in fights. That's actually how cutman Jacob 'Stitch' Duran and I became such good friends. I would always be in Marcus's corner and knew we would be needing the services of a cutman. I knew we would need some good cut work and preventative work with things such as the enswell [a handheld, curved metal compression block that helps compress the hematoma to help with swelling]. Most people don't realize that before entering MMA, Davis had close to 100 boxing matches where he had built up a lot of scar tissue. We knew he would get cut in a fight."

It's important fighters know that facial lacerations don't just affect the match you're fighting in the Octagon, but that the consequences could be long term. When scar tissue builds up cut after cut, even punches during practice could prove damaging. As DellaGrotte explains, "During our training camps for [Marcus] Davis, we would have him wear big *Battlestar Galactica*–like headgear. His training partners would use 18 oz gloves instead of 16 oz gloves for extra padding. Everyone had to be bundled up like a little kid in winter to prevent additional damage, some of which could prevent him from being able to fight in his next bout."

## ANATOMY

Besides knockouts and submissions, significant cuts and bleeding are common reasons for a fight to be stopped. They are also the reason why skilled cutmen are sought after. Despite weeks or months of training, a bad cut can stop a fight as quickly as an unseen right hook or a rear naked choke. Fortunately, the long-term effects of most cuts are considerably less than the drama they create during a bout. Unless they are in certain high-risk areas, which we will examine later, it is rare for a cut to have any serious functional consequences after the fight. However, if you do accumulate a lot of scar tissue from repeated cuts and bleeding, you may end up becoming a fighter that bleeds more easily in a fight.

Cuts occur through the direct transfer of energy from a strike, which is usually absorbed by the harder bony structures. However, the skin and subcutaneous (under the skin) structures are often caught in the middle and can be damaged either by being crushed in the energy "blast" such as in a head-butt or by being sheared as a glove moves across the skin. In essence, the skin is spread apart as the underlying bone pushes out against the soft tissue. Sometimes, the visible cut is just the tip of the iceberg.

### THE TWO TYPES OF BLEEDING

Bleeding can be classified as arterial or venous. Arterial bleeding results from damage to arteries, which are the vessels in the outflow track from the heart and thus have a pulsatile quality and can bleed in greater quantities more quickly. During a fight, you may see the distinct droplet spray-pattern on the canvas of an arterial bleed. Venous bleeding occurs when veins are damaged. Veins are the vessels that return the blood to the heart and therefore are under less pressure. Venous bleeds are often slower and non-pulsatile. These appear more as a long drip coming off the fighter's nose or a pool on the canvas. Some areas of the face are more prone to serious injuries than others. Legendary boxing and MMA cutman Jacob "Stitch" Duran likes to point out one area in particular that causes a lot of bleeding: "That big vein that we all have between our eyes; when they pop that one, I know that I've got my job cut out."

## DANGER ZONES AND REASONS TO STOP A FIGHT

Cuts around the eyebrow can cause bleeding that affects a fighter's vision and ability to protect themself. They can also damage important nerves. If the cut is deep enough above the eyebrow, it can lead to damage of the supraorbital nerve. The same can be said for below the eye, where the infraorbital nerve lies. These nerves supply feeling from the skin near the top of the head down to the upper eyelid and from the upper lip to the lower eyelid, respectively. A cut on the actual eyelid always has a risk of being particularly dangerous to underlying structures. An important structure called the nasolacrimal duct runs from the area between the eye and the nose to just under the eye. If this area is damaged, the normal ability for tears to hydrate the eye can be inhibited, leading to significant long-term eyes issues. And remember, if the cut is severe enough for a ringside doctor to stop a fight, it certainly should be enough to stop a sparring match during training.

Some of the reasons a ringside physician may stop a fight due to a cut include:

1. Significant arterial bleeding resulting in rapid and continuing blood loss.
2. Exposure of underlying nerves or bone (including broken bones).
3. Vision impairment. A cut may affect a fighter's vision, either from bleeding or the location of the laceration.
4. The location of the cut. The eyelid and the eye area near the nose are high-risk areas and can result in irreparable damage.

Stitch has seen how lacerations can stop fights and knows that if you can't stop the bleeding, then the fight should be over. "If it's a real big, old, nasty, gnarly cut that's above the eyebrow or something that may get you into nerve-damage territory, then it might be time to call it. But it's usually more a case of blood getting into a fighter's eye more than anything else. If you work on it for that one minute you get between rounds and he goes out and right off the bat it's gushing blood again, and it's going into his eyes and he's starting to wipe his eyes, and you give it another shot and it's just not working, then it might be time to go ahead and call that a night for the fighter, so he can come back the next day."

Do any cuts stick out in Stitch's mind? There is one story he likes to tell. "When BJ Penn fought Joe Stevenson, we were in England at *UFC 80*. I was working BJ Penn's corner and Joe Stevenson ended up with a big gash between his eyes. He was bleeding like a pig and they stopped the fight. As cutmen, we get assigned to a specific corner for the night. Back in the dressing room, Joe kept asking, 'Where was Stitch? Where's Stitch?' You see, those guys look up to what we do as cutmen. I think, especially of all the cutmen, they have a lot of confidence in me and that was just a nice little gesture. It was nice that he made that kind of comment."


## TREATMENT

Compression is the cutman's best friend. Stitch will tell you, the easiest method to reduce bleeding of any kind, including lacerations, is simple pressure. Applying gauze and pressure is the most reliable method to allow the blood to clot and reduce blood flow out of the wound. The reason behind this is that if blood is flowing, it can't begin the process of solidifying into a clot. Compression helps stabilize the blood flow and allows the blood to coagulate, which prevents further bleeding. The enswell is an example of a device cutmen can use to help compress bleeding wounds to encourage clotting, but not all cutmen are using these devices properly. As Stitch explains, "I also see a lot of the guys working with the enswells trying to move the hematoma [a pocket of clotted blood under the skin] around. In fact, as I was coming up through the ranks I was told to get that clot and try to move it to the side. But talking with the ringside doctors now that know the business, what you're doing is just moving that blood into tissue that is not damaged. And it eventually comes right back. So direct pressure with a cold compress closes up most blood vessels, and that's really the basic principle we work with. Compression is what guys are doing right."

Some cutmen will employ epinephrine (adrenaline), which is a medicine that causes blood vessels to constrict and thus limit how much blood can flow out. This often requires a prescription and the legal use of it varies by jurisdiction. They may mix it with Vaseline and put it on a fighter's face between rounds. Other compounds that can reduce blood flow include seaweed extracts and synthetic thrombin, which is a chemical in the blood-clotting process. Many fighters have also described using store-bought superglue, but this practice cannot be endorsed as safe by any medical professional.

Stitch also notes that one thing that may make bleeding worse is taking anti-inflammatories, as they may increase the risk for bleeding. Aspirin and anti-inflammatories such as ibuprofen have a theoretical disadvantage in that they may reduce the blood's efficiency in clotting. "One of the things that I always ask the guys is what kind of medications they're on and if they are taking any anti-inflammatories. When they get banged up, I know that'll make my job a little bit harder."

Both prevention and good work by cutmen during a bout are important. Mark DellaGrotte, one of the UFC's top trainers, recalls one fight he was cornering that sticks out in his mind, "Joe Lauzon versus Mac Danzig. In rounds 1 to 2, Joe got a large hematoma, like a potato, and came back lumped up and swollen. Rather than use the enswell, they send him back out with a big hematoma and he gets cut there and starts to bleed. Just because there aren't cuts actively bleeding doesn't mean that you can't use things like the enswell or Vaseline to prevent the cut from happening or getting worse."

If a laceration is deep enough, it will need to be stitched, which should occur in the hands of a trained physician. The skin has several layers to it, and a suture job that seeks to close a very deep, jagged wound to merely stop the bleeding, and doesn't address the underlying layers, may result in skin that is scarred and less strong than skin that is properly repaired and healed. Several prominent fighters have sought out plastic surgeons to help them deal with the years of scar tissue that have built up under their skin from years of cuts.

Nick Diaz's coach Cesar Gracie has battled with Nick's cuts and sought out such treatment. "Nick's biggest problem was getting cut. Nick has very sharp bones on his eyebrows so he gets cut very easily. The bone pushes on the skin from the inside. He actually had plastic surgery in Las Vegas to grind down the bone."

Deciding when to return to contact training depends on where the laceration is in the healing process. Normal skin follows a regular pattern for healing. At two weeks, the skin is about 20% as strong as its pre-injury level. By five weeks, it is about 50% healed. By 10 weeks, it is about 80% of pre-injury strength and may stay at that level forever. It is a safe bet to say that a minimum of six weeks is required before a significantly deep laceration is healed enough for the fighter to return to sparring. If it was a particularly deep cut, up to three months may be required before full contact resumes.

## PREVENTING INFECTION

One of the primary functions of skin is to prevent infections. A break in the skin means a risk for bacteria to invade and create an infection, which can rapidly get out of control. Sometimes they can lead to the well-known staph infection. Stitch, cutman for both the UFC and boxing's world-champion Klitschko brothers, remarks on how important keeping wounds clean is to the health of a fighter: "Right now I look at a lot of the cutmen out there and the first thing I always do is tell those guys that the swabs we use to apply epine [short for epinephrine] on the cut need to stay clean. You'll see these cutmen put the swabs in the fighter's mouths and they put them in their ears. And the first thing I tell them is to keep them sanitary and watch where they put them."

The most effective way to prevent infection after a cut is to keep the injury site as clean as possible. Although it may seem as though fixing cuts is a cosmetic procedure, there could be serious consequences should an infection appear. In Dean Lister's experience, care should be taken both before and after a laceration occurs: "To help prevent cuts before sparring hard, you need to Vaseline the high-risk areas thoroughly, especially around the ridges of the eyebrows and under the eyes where the cuts are most likely to occur. After receiving a cut, which happens in MMA and boxing of course, please seek medical attention, especially if stitches are needed. After that, you will probably get more attention from the ladies! But most importantly, keep the threat of infection to a minimum and be sure to keep the area very clean." Neosporin is one over-the-counter option that has both anti-bacterial and anti-fungal medications. It is good to keep a healing laceration covered if it's in an area where it will be rubbed a lot, such as by clothing. And don't forget the effectiveness of simple soap and water for keeping the bacteria away! As we will see later in the book, skin infections can have serious consequences.

## INJURY PREVENTION

### HEADGEAR AND VASELINE – ADVICE FROM THE PROS

As Mark DellaGrotte points out, wearing appropriate padding during training can help lengthen your career by reducing the amount of trauma and facial injury that builds up. UFC champion Sean "The Muscle Shark" Sherk also understands the importance of preventing lacerations, not just during fights but also in training. Sometimes the danger is worse if the guy you are training with isn't well trained. "My worst cut I can remember was from a knee when I shot in on a guy during a training camp. I ended up needing to miss my fight 10 days after. I needed 60 stitches. In fact, I get cut under the chin a lot — as most wrestlers do. I would even have to duct tape it. My advice is be careful who you train with. Your injury risk probably triples when guys are hacks and don't know what they are doing. And wear headgear. I know you can't hide your whole body, and you need to know what it's like to feel a hard shot, but you also need to be smart and protect yourself!"

When it comes to preventing cuts, Cesar Gracie points to headgear: "I have noticed that kickboxers at my academy don't like headgear, but for boxers, it's natural and they always use it, so it's an interesting combo in MMA. For the guys that don't want to wear it, I remind them that their livelihood is fighting. If you get cut and have to pull out of the fight, it's going to come out of your pocket. If you want to be a professional, you need to wear headgear. I also always apply Vaseline to my fighters. And more importantly, make sure to check and reapply every two to three rounds."

Don Frye has had two significant lacerations that he can remember, and he has his own tips for fighters that seem to come straight from working on a ranch. "During the *Ultimate Ultimate 2* in 1996, Tank Abbott busted my eye to the bone in the finals. I have had that same eye split open with a head-butt against another guy. My advice to avoid getting cut? Make sure to use Vaseline. Maybe even use some butter balm to soften the skin like we do with cows. When you train for a long time on the mats, your feet become dry and cracked and this stuff can help moisten them, too. It helps get you back in the saddle."

Headgear during training not only protects from hand strikes, but also from inadvertent head-butts. UFC champion Matt Serra, the only man to knock out Georges St-Pierre, has had some experience with inadvertent head-butts. "In the last fight of my career, in the opening round, I was throwing some hands against Chris Lytle. We crashed heads and I got head-butted. I needed a bunch of stitches. Head-butts are dangerous and should be avoided in training. When training, even if it's just wrestling, at least one guy needs to wear headgear to prevent head-butts. They can really cut people open."

Padded protection shouldn't just be limited to the head. In the Octagon, UFC champion Jon Jones is known for his devastating elbows, which can slice open an opponent in the blink of an eye. Jones practices these strikes with an elbow routine under the supervision of Greg Jackson and Mike Winkeljohn. Because elbows can be so dangerous, Jon wears elbow pads while sparring. "Jon is good enough where he can actually just tap a guy with his elbow, but even he wears pads while training. It protects him, his training partners, and our team. All guys should use them," says Winkeljohn.

Coach and former UFC champion Josh Barnett also sees elbows as especially dangerous during training. "To avoid cuts, I don't allow anyone to throw elbows unless they have nice secured elbow pads, and then they are allowed to just touch their partner. No hammering. If you can't avoid hammering them, you don't have the skill. If I can't control my opponent and then perform the finishing strike without

**SUMMARY OF ZONES**

1. tarsal plate, lacrimal sac
2. vermilion border
3. supraorbital/ supratrochlear nerves
4. nasal bridge
5. infraorbital nerve
6. nasolabial fold with facial artery
7. superficial temporal artery, facial nerve (at the zygomatic bone)
8. facial artery at masseter
9. mental nerve

ZONES OF CONCERN FOR LACERATIONS. GRAY MEANS WATCH CLOSELY DURING A FIGHT AND DARK GRAY MEANS STOP THE FIGHT.

hurting them, then I need to work on that technique. If you do get cut, give it time to heal. I know it sucks sitting on the sideline, but you can do other things so it doesn't get opened back up."

## CHAPTER 3

# EYE INJURIES AND
# ORBITAL FRACTURES

## ANATOMY

UFC and MMA veteran light heavyweight Brandon Vera has had some scary moments with facial injuries, including one significant orbital fracture. "After my fight with Randy Couture, I fought Jon Jones. I had a tripod orbital fracture on the right side of my face, which I received from one of Jon Jones's elbows. A piece of bone went behind my eye and I had to have significant reconstruction surgery. To this day, it's my worst injury — pain-wise and in terms of recovery. The injury was so severe that the doctors worried whether I would have vision in that eye, and I worried about when I would fight again. During my next fight, with Thiago Silva, I broke my nose from a hook while on the ground. I couldn't get the juice monkey off of me. I noticed it right after my fight, while looking on the camera. I remember looking at it and thinking, 'Holy shit, I hope the doctors can put it back together and make me good-looking again.' It was actually a blessing in disguise. My whole life I had a deviated septum. I never understood when people said breathe through your nose until after my surgery and healing process. I could now finally breathe through my nose. To date that was my third most painful surgery, and I had to have my nose fixed. I don't understand how people get that done as an elective procedure!"

Eye injuries in MMA typically fall under two main categories: abrasions and blunt trauma. Abrasions usually occur when the eye is scratched by a fingernail, a toe, or even a glove. The cornea is the clear portion that covers the center of the eye. When the cornea is injured, it feels like a sharp pain and often gives the sensation that there is something in the eye. Doctors are usually able to diagnose this by putting a special dye into the eye and seeing if a scratch or tear appears bright with a special fluorescent light. Because the pain is often so bad and even bright lights cause the eye to want to close, it would be very difficult for a fighter to adequately defend himself after this occurs. Treatment is usually with antibiotic drops to prevent infection, but this requires seeing a doctor. If a fighter fails to see a doctor, and the eye gets infected, a minor scratch can became a nightmare. Treated appropriately, minor scratches can heal in just a couple of days. Larger abrasions may take a little longer.

Sometimes, bleeding can actually happen inside the eye itself. When this happens, a layer of blood inside the eyeball may cover some of the iris and the pupil. This is called hyphema. Treatment usually consists of preventing further bleeding, such as bed rest with the head of the bed elevated. Often these bleeds are small and resolve on their own, but sometimes they can progress and this can lead to permanent vision problems, including glaucoma. Anti-inflammatories may increase a fighter's risk of further bleeding and should be avoided in this injury.

The more serious eye injuries may come from blunt trauma. The major part of the eye is a fluid-filled oval structure known as the globe. With compression of the globe, the retina or optic nerve at the back of the eye may be injured or torn. The eye focuses light on the retina similarly to how a camera focuses light onto a sensor. The retina translates that focused image into nerve impulses and sends them to the brain via the optic nerve. If the retina is damaged, the fighter may see flashes of light, or "floaters." If it tears completely, a person could become blind. Therefore, if a fighter starts to see these "floaters," no matter what stage of his career, he should see an eye doctor. With enough force applied to the eye, the globe itself can actually rupture. This usually results in pain, vision loss, or even leakage of the fluid within the globe. This type of injury often requires prompt evaluation by an ophthalmologist (eye doctor). This can be a surgical emergency. Thus, a fighter and his trainer should be familiar with these signs of serious injury.

---

**PAT MILETICH'S THREE COMPONENTS TO MAKE TRAINING AND FIGHTING SAFER**

1. Staying in shape, both anaerobic and aerobic
2. Flexibility
3. Coaches paying attention to fatigue and keeping fighters moving in good form

---

## ORBITAL FRACTURES

If the blunt force is strong enough, the orbital bones or other bones that are near the eye can fracture (which is the same as a break). It was at *UFC 10*, which marked the UFC's return to a format featuring an eight-man tournament, that Don "The Predator" Frye suffered his most significant facial fracture against Mark "The Hammer" Coleman. "During *UFC 10*, Mark Coleman broke my orbital. I remember waking up that day feeling sick, but I kept fighting the whole time. I certainly put myself at risk. When you're an athlete and in tune with your body, you know something is wrong, and I knew it.

"My first fight was against Mark Hall. I wore myself out with him. I went for the ribs instead of head and tired myself out. Then in my second bout of the night, I fought judo black belt and Golden Gloves winner Brian Johnston. He is a powerful guy and kicked me hard a couple times. I thought I might need to quit, but I managed to win the fight. Backstage after the fight, my trainer Steve Owen saw I was completely tired and dehydrated. We discussed pulling out of the finals against Mark Coleman. But I sat in that chair and I looked around at the alternates. I thought to myself there is no way

I would send these kids in to the lions, to face Mark Coleman. So I went in there to take my beating."

UFC veteran Nick Diaz also suffered an orbital fracture. His coach Cesar Gracie recalls the story, "Nick had an orbital fracture. We think it probably got broken against Gomi in Pride. We never got any x-rays at the time, but he had a lot of bruising. After another fight, he got x-rays and they saw the fracture. He had to let it heal with time. Sensitivity was our guide. Anytime someone has a face fracture, we make sure to use masks. We have masks for training, especially for broken noses. The ones we use are not bulky like boxing but slimmer for MMA. If the fighter needs to stay busy during the healing process, we put headgear on, plus a mask."

As mentioned before, elbows are especially dangerous around the face. They can open up big cuts, but the focused force can also cause a facial fracture. UFC Welterweight Champion Carlos Newton felt firsthand what it's like to have a broken facial bone from an elbow blow. "In the first round of my fight with Charuto at *UFC 46*, he threw a funny punch during a ground-and-pound and I felt a pop in my cheek. After my decision loss, the ringside doctor saw me. I felt okay and looked okay to him. But as it turned out, I probably ended up breaking my orbital bone. The broken bone formed a bump when it healed, which created a point that leads to bruising and easy cutting. Of course, this led me to develop a better skill of not getting hit in the face. . . . When it comes to face injuries, you really need to watch out for elbows. They can generate enough force and the bone comes to a point, which easily causes injury like orbital fractures. I always found it interesting that in Japan, where they have very competitive rules, despite being able to kick a guy while he was down like in Pride, we couldn't throw elbows. What is also dangerous is that orbital fractures don't usually end a fight and can get overlooked."

## INJURY PREVENTION

Ninety percent of eye injuries in other sports can be prevented with eye protection; unfortunately, this is not possible in MMA.

Other than a physical barrier, there isn't anything anyone can do to "strengthen" the eye against injury. Top striking coach Mike Winkeljohn has personally felt the effects of getting poked in the eye by a kick, and the consequence was serious. "I was holding pads and not paying attention and got a toenail to my eye, injuring my globe. I asked the person that kicked me if I was cut. He goes, 'No, coach, it's your eyeball.' I felt moisture, and it was all the fluid from inside my eye. It just shriveled up like a little grape. I was in shock, so I didn't feel it. I saw my doctor's face after she examined me and knew something was bad. I underwent four surgeries before the optic nerve died and I lost vision out of that eye."

Cesar Gracie has noticed two things that can prevent eye pokes. "In training, most guys use the 6–8 oz gloves, so it's harder to straighten your fingers, but when they step in the cage with the 4 oz gloves, they straighten their fingers and that can lead to more eye pokes in the cage. The other thing guys can do is keep fingernails and toenails clipped. In kickboxing especially, the feet and toes are exposed under the pads and can lead to eye pokes."

Like most aspects of training, using the right equipment for training exercises is important. Traditional boxing gloves are mostly rounded and the fingers are contained, reducing the incidence of eye pokes. MMA gloves, however, allow the fingers to be exposed, which is crucial for grappling. Furthermore, MMA often involves unorthodox striking, including open hand or overhand strikes that can easily result in a thumb to the eye. UFC Hall of Famer Pat Miletich understands there is a balance between using MMA gloves for grappling, but boxing gloves for striking. He makes sure his fighters always wear boxing gloves when striking, both for safety and technique. "Guys with MMA gloves develop bad habits like not hitting fully and leaning back to avoid fingers coming into eyes. I have my guys use MMA gloves for grappling technique in the morning but full boxing gloves at night for striking practice."

MMA is a sport where injuries can easily happen. It is the job of everyone involved, from the trainers and fighters to the referees and ringside physicians, to do what they can to help prevent injuries.

However, when injuries do occur, and they will, the team needs to do what's best for the fighter. If there are any signs of eye damage, the fight or training session should be stopped. Not being able to see out of an eye puts the fighter at risk of further damage. If a fighter does lose sight in one eye, he will be hard-pressed to find a commission or doctor who would ever let him fight again.

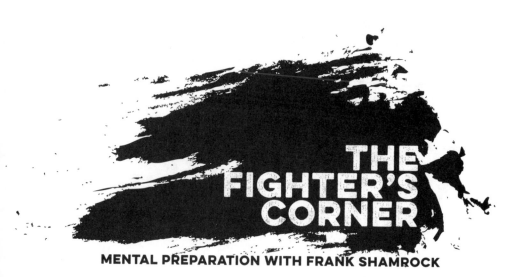

# THE FIGHTER'S CORNER

**MENTAL PREPARATION WITH FRANK SHAMROCK**

Many fighters focus on preserving their body, but they should also focus on preserving their mind. The biggest key to successful combat and competition is complete mental preparation. So, what is mental preparation and how do you train your mind?

Most sporting competitions come down to decisions made in milliseconds by your body. Other times you may have to react without even making a conscious thought. This quick reaction is accomplished from training. The body and the mind need to work in unison. Your mind is a supercomputer able to compute under extreme stress, but when the mind is not prepared, it becomes consumed with fear and other distractive information. Training the mind is as, if not more, important as physical training. When you train in martial arts or competitive sports, you are wiring your brain and your body to interact and react together.

There are several tools one can employ to create a strong mental preparation routine for MMA. The first tool is visualization. Visualization is a broad term that sports psychologists

---

**FRANK SHAMROCK'S
TOP THREE POINTS FOR
INJURY PREVENTION**

1. Strengthening
2. Stretching
3. Icing

---

use to describe techniques where we imagine ourselves performing sport-specific tasks, including what we feel, see, hear, and touch. This helps establish a routine and also prepare us for the situations that may arise in competition. By "experiencing" these moments beforehand, we can react quicker and more predictably when the actual situation arises. In truth, most of us visualize already, but we fill our minds with daydreams of what we wish our life to be. This is not true, focused visualization training. Actual mental training takes practice and patience and focuses on a specific goal.

For example, with grappling, I visualize performing each technique and how each technique flows to the next and how those techniques tie together to accomplish my goal of submitting my opponent. This can apply to any practiced movements with your body that you can visualize in your mind — golf, baseball, boxing, even playing music.

You may notice during your visualization training that your heart rate may elevate or your body may tense. This is the mind connecting to your body. The ability to control this stimulation can be found with quiet breathing exercises and meditation. If we return to the brain-as-supercomputer analogy, meditation is the time to defragment your hard drive and reboot back up with new, cleanly organized information. Meditation complements the physical training process by relaxing the body and clearing doubts, fears, and other confusing thoughts. During meditation you can slow your thoughts, relax your mind, and begin to analyze any anxieties or fears you may have. I even use it before broadcast announcing where I know my face will be in front of millions of people watching at home.

Finally, the third component of proper mental preparation is focusing on slow, controlled physical movement. Physical forms such as yoga, t'ai chi, or shadowboxing are all techniques that can help wire the body and mind together in a controlled and relaxed environment. This helps you focus on keeping good form for when you go full speed.

Through the use of these three tools — visualization, meditation, and slow physical forms — you will be able to perform at your peak during MMA competition. When people say it's all in your mind, they are exactly right.

## CHAPTER **4**
# KNEE INJURIES AND RETURNING
# TO THE OCTAGON AFTER SURGERY

When an athlete has a significant knee injury, whole sports worlds can change. A team can lose their star player for the season. An entire UFC card can be canceled because the headliner was injured. Or the reigning, dominant champion can be knocked out of competition for over a year. One of the most talked about knee injuries in MMA occurred in 2011. While preparing for a fight against Carlos Condit, Georges St-Pierre defended a wrestling takedown attempt by his training partner and felt a pop in his right knee. For weeks prior he had been compensating for other seemingly minor injuries, especially in his right knee, but in this instance it became clear the pop he felt was serious. There was not much swelling on the knee initially, so he tried to continue training. However, he soon found it was difficult for him to walk normally and in the few days afterwards, he continued to feel pain as well as instability. He called his doctor, who suggested he get an MRI in Las Vegas. The MRI revealed he suffered from a torn ACL in his right knee that would require surgery. This injury put the champion out of action for the better part of a year. Most critics felt he would never return to championship form. After all, the list of running backs in the NFL that never returned to the same level of performance after an ACL rupture was ever growing. However, proving that he truly is a champion, GSP had surgery, rehabbed his knee, and went on to defeat then–interim champion Carlos Condit by unanimous decision after a grueling five-round 25-minute bout. As we will see later, Condit had his own experience with an ACL Injury, and St-Pierre's experience provided him with some advice.

## ANATOMY

Understanding the anatomy of the knee is important to understanding its injuries. The knee is composed of the femur (thigh bone), tibia (shin bone), and patella (kneecap). As the connection between the femur and tibia, the knee acts as a hinge allowing the leg to bend. The knee can experience considerable stress when changing levels and shooting in for a takedown, snapping a kick, or quickly moving out of the way of an opponent's attack.

The femur has two rounded ends that rest on top of the tibia. Since the top of the tibia is relatively flat, the body has adapted to create two semi-circular cushions of cartilage called the menisci (plural for meniscus). The menisci help the femur fit into the tibia as well as provide stability and act as shock absorbers in the knee, distributing force and protecting the surface cartilage from damage.

The knee is also held in place by several ligaments. Ligaments are soft-tissue structures that run from one bone to another. This is in contrast to tendons, which are the ends of muscles that thicken and insert into bones to allow them to pull. Within the center of the knee are two ligaments that cross each other ("cruciate" meaning crossing). The ACL, or anterior (front) cruciate ligament, lies in front, and the PCL, or posterior (back) cruciate ligament, lies in the back. On the inner side of the knee running from the femur to the tibia is the MCL, medial collateral ligament, and on the outer side of the knee running from the femur to the fibula is the LCL, lateral collateral ligament.

## ACL INJURIES

*Ultimate Fighter 3* finalist Ed Herman knows firsthand what it feels like to rupture his ACL in the Octagon. During his *UFC 102* bout against All-American wrestler Aaron Simpson, his knee was forced backwards into an awkward position. "Simpson shot a double leg and then I felt instant pain. It hurt like hell. I didn't realize how bad it was, so I continued to fight and tried to answer the bell in the second round. When I came out to fight, I threw a kick and there was nothing there underneath me. My knee just buckled. At first, there was almost no swelling, so I thought I sprained it. But then I saw the doctor and we got an MRI. It showed I had torn my ACL."

### HOW THE ACL TEARS

The ACL acts to prevent the tibia from moving forward away from the femur and helps prevent the knee from buckling during sudden changes in direction such as cutting, twisting, or even kicking. The ACL can be injured when one part of the knee suddenly rotates quicker than the other, such as when it is grabbed and twisted during grappling or when a fighter quickly pivots with a planted foot to kick or change direction. In addition, the ACL can also be injured when a fighter's knee is hit from the side, similar to when a football player hits someone's knee during a tackle. In fact, since MMA has so many facets, the injuries an MMA fighter sees arches across many sports. ACL injuries are more common in sports such as football where players often need to suddenly stop and change direction, but these injuries commonly strike MMA fighters as well. Baseball players or other overhead athletes often injure their shoulders through overuse injuries, yet MMA fighters injure their shoulders and rotator cuffs as well.

Carlos Condit had a common injury mechanism during his *UFC 171* co–main event bout against Tyron Woodley. "In the second round of the fight, I tore my ACL and both menisci. During the round I stepped wrong, and I felt a pretty intense burning and could feel the sensation that my bones shifted. I went down to the guard,

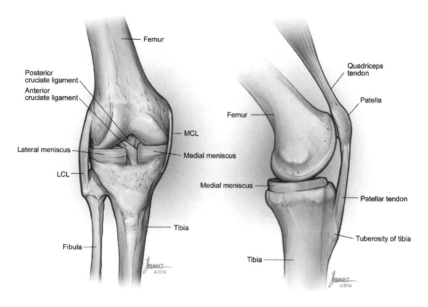

FRONT AND SIDE VIEWS OF THE KNEE WITH LIGAMENTS AND MENISCI SHOWN. CREDIT: JOE KANASZ.

the pain improved, and we stood back up. Then, he kicked my other knee from the outside. I went to pivot on the injured knee and my whole knee gave out."

## ACL RECONSTRUCTION

Like all ligaments, the ACL can either be sprained (partial tear) or ruptured (completely torn). When the ACL is ruptured, the athlete may often hear a "pop" and then experience quick pain and swelling of the knee. They can tell pretty soon something is wrong with their knee and will feel a sense of instability. Complete tears will require surgery to continue participating in sports that require sudden directional changes. A complete tear of the ACL cannot heal on its own, so the surgery is referred to as an ACL "reconstruction," which means replacing it with a new ACL graft. Different surgeons and different athletes prefer different types of grafts to reconstruct the ACL. Georges St-Pierre underwent reconstruction with his own patellar tendon graft.

Cat Zingano, a top female MMA athlete used a cadaver graft. UFC Bantamweight Champion Dominick Cruz had a cadaver graft for his initial surgery and then used his own patellar tendon for his second ACL surgery on the same knee. Ed Herman used his own hamstring graft for his first surgery and a cadaver patellar tendon for the second.

Deciding which ACL graft to use is a topic that has been, and will likely continue to be, hotly debated by surgeons. Large-scale studies have shown that there is likely no difference in re-tear rates between your own hamstring and patellar tendon grafts, but both of these tend to do better than cadaver grafts since they are your own tissue. You can feel your patellar tendon if you bend your knee and feel the front of your leg, just below your kneecap. When a patellar tendon graft is used, a piece of bone is taken out of the patella and another piece is taken from your tibia with a strand of patellar tendon in between. This graft is thought to have the best chance of healing, since it has bone on the ends, which the hamstring graft does not. Unfortunately, a side effect may be pain when kneeling down, something grapplers do all the time. There may also be some weakness in the quadriceps, the muscles that straighten your leg, which could weaken the "snap" of your kick. The potential for kneeling pain is why Herman decided on a hamstring graft with his surgeon. "I didn't want to use my own patella tendon because my surgeon said there was a risk of sensitivity in the front of the knee and [I could have] trouble kneeling." The hamstring graft is taken where some of the hamstring tendons wrap around to the front of the knee. The benefit of using a hamstring graft instead of a patellar tendon graft is that the pain of having to take bone with the graft and the subsequent kneeling pain is eliminated. The theoretical downsides are that there is no bone on the ends of the graft for healing into the femur and tibia bones directly and you may lose some of your knee flexion (bending) strength.

The third option is to use a cadaver ligament. This method avoids all the pain of harvesting the graft from your own body (which can be the most painful part of the surgery) and may make your rehab easier. The downside is that there is a risk of disease transmission, although this is significantly lower than in past decades. Since it's not your own tissue, it may not be the best choice for a younger, elite athlete and some studies have shown it can be four times more likely to fail. However, in Ed Herman's case, since he already used his hamstring from the injured knee as a graft the first time around, he and his surgeon chose to use a cadaver tendon for the second surgery.

## PRE-HAB, REHAB, AND GETTING BACK TO 100%

It's not only the fighters who are at risk for an ACL rupture in the Octagon. The "Veteran Voice of the Octagon" Bruce Buffer is an announcer known for his exciting spins during his introduction of fighters. At *UFC 129* in Toronto, with 55,000 people in the stands, Buffer was getting ready to announce Canadian Georges St-Pierre in front of one of the largest crowds in UFC history. GSP was standing a few feet away, ready to face off against Jake Shields in front of a largely Canadian crowd. Buffer started like he normally does with his trademark "It's time!" catchphrase and an introduction of Shields, but he really reached deep to announce the name of GSP. Suddenly, GSP bounced forward towards him in excitement and Buffer had to hop back abruptly. This sudden change in direction led to Buffer tearing his ACL.

Buffer is the UFC's top announcer and has a mind-blowing travel schedule. He delayed his surgery until his schedule allowed him some time off, and in the interim focused on getting his body ready for surgery. He knew he needed to work on not only his post-surgery rehab, but also his pre-surgery "pre-hab." Bruce recalls, "When I booked my operation a few months ahead of time due to my appearance schedule, my trainer and I trained the leg intensively to make it as strong as possible for my ACL operation and it worked to make a very healthy environment for my doctor to replace my ACL. I even went off pain medication the day after and rehabbed quickly, which I attest to the physical shape I was in going into the operating room." Focusing on ACL pre-hab is a great way to get ready for an upcoming ACL surgery.

After surgery, the final thing you must face is your post-operative rehabilitation. ACL rehab is not easy and usually takes at least six months, and it will most likely take up to a year until you are feeling close to 100%. Working on your range of motion is one of the first things you will do, then you will begin to focus on your hamstrings, and then work your way up to your quadriceps. The quadriceps are the first to weaken, even before surgery, so it's important to keep your quadriceps strong before and after your surgery.

Ed Herman knew if he wanted to get back to the UFC, he needed to really focus on his rehab. "I did some intensive rehab. It was hard. I started the day after surgery and was there five days a week. My advice to other fighters recovering from ACL surgery is to hit the rehab hard, but make sure to do it with professionals. And don't force it. Don't try and come back to wrestling and sparring too soon."

Ed brings up a very important topic. Despite excellent outcomes from ACL surgeries, many athletes who have already had an ACL tear will experience another one. A systematic review of studies has shown that within five years of surgery, about 6% of athletes will tear their same ACL and around 12% will tear their other ACL.[1] Three years after returning to championship form from his ACL tear, GSP tore the ACL in his other knee. Three months after his ACL surgery, Ed Herman tore his newly reconstructed ACL. Many of these re-tears within the first year happen because the athlete isn't fully rehabbed from their knee surgery. Often, they are still favoring their other knee and have limited balance on their operative knee. In fact, one study showed there is an equal (3%) chance of tearing the ACL in either the reconstructed or the "good" knee within just two years of surgery.[2]

Ed recalls his second injury, "When I re-tore it, it was only three

---

1 "Ipsilateral Graft and Contralateral ACL Rupture at Five Years or More Following ACL Reconstruction: A Systematic Review." Wright RW, Magnussen RA, Dunn WR, Spindler KP. *J Bone Joint Surg Am.* 2011 Jun 15; 93(12): 1159–65

2 "Risk of Tearing the Intact Anterior Cruciate Ligament in the Contralateral Knee and Rupturing the Anterior Cruciate Ligament Graft During the First 2 Years After Anterior Cruciate Ligament Reconstruction: A Prospective MOON Cohort Study." Wright RW. *Am J Sports Med.* 2007 Jul; 35(7): 1131–4

months after surgery. I tried to come back too soon. I think I was cleared to do light training. I was further along than anyone at my rehab place had ever seen that soon after surgery. But then again, they aren't used to dealing with professional athletes. I was doing a skip knee drill. I was holding my training partner's head in a Thai plum clinch, alternating knees with a light jumping motion to his chest. I came down on the outside of my foot on the soft mats, and boom! I knew I re-tore it right away." MMA athletes are known for their determination and perseverance. There is no off-season to recover like other sports, so the fighter is often very eager to return to competition, always pushing the boundaries. But it's important, especially with a big surgery like ACL reconstruction, to give yourself the full recovery time, even if it takes more than a year. The risk of a second surgery, being out even longer, and making your knee worse is not worth the risk of dangerously shortening your rehab period.

UFC Hall of Famer Mark Coleman suffered his first MMA injury at age 31. "[It] was an ACL tear in my right knee. My right knee is my lead knee, which may have made it more susceptible to injury. In 1997, I was 31. I had just won the UFC title in 1996. I had many injuries in wrestling, but nothing that required surgery. I got stuck up in the corner, and a guy put his shoulder in me, and my knee went out. I knew it was a big one. I was out for eight months. Back in 1996, they were getting better with ACL surgery, and I had serious atrophy versus now when they get you moving right away. My first fight was five months later against Pete Williams, and I am not going to blame the loss on my ACL, but my leg was definitely not ready. Back then I was my own coach. I probably should not have taken the fight and it was not a good evening for me. Athletes have an itch. They want to get back in there quickly. And some do, but many end up back on the sideline. Athletes often are strong headed, but they need to listen to their coaches and their doctors. If you want to be wise, you rehab your knee and you get back in there when you are truly ready."

Patrick Côté underwent ACL surgery and it took him over a year to get back, which is not unexpected. "I had my ACL reconstruction in 2009. It took me a year and a half to be ready to get back in competition. My doc did an amazing job, but it takes time to heal both physically and mentally. Now my knee is 100%." Patrick brings up another excellent point — a fighter also needs to consider the amount of time it takes to mentally heal from ACL reconstruction. This type of recovery has been shown to be just as important, as some athletes never return to their sport simply out of fear of re-injury. Like most of these athletes, it took UFC veteran and U.S. Army Ranger Tim Kennedy one year to feel fully recovered from his ACL surgery. But he has some advice on how to tell when you are truly recovered and ready to push it. "I tore my ACL wrestling in college and had surgery. At seven months out, I was in the army and jumping out of airplanes, but it took one year until I felt right. I was very disciplined in my rehab and then carried that through my career and continue to strongly focus on injury prevention. Part of coming back from an injury is being mentally ready to push yourself. Until you are dripping sweat and crying from just your workout and forgetting about your leg, that's when it's time to really train — when you can forget about surgery and your injury, when you have rehabbed fully, have confidence in your recovery, and forget what it's like to be afraid."

After the surgery, sticking to a well-thought-out, guided physical therapy program is the next step in making sure you have a good outcome from ACL reconstructions. Ed points out the importance of working with good physical therapists during your recovery: "Make sure your rehab is guided by professionals who specialize in ACL or other sports surgical rehab. They, along with your surgeon, will help guide you back to where you need to be to get back to fighting." Tim Kennedy agrees, "If you can, seek out a sports-specific physical therapist who understands your sport. Before you see the physical therapist, see who he has worked with, where he has learned and worked before. Is he known in your sport and your community? Talk to your doctors about who they recommend."

When Carlos Condit ruptured his ACL, his former opponent Georges St-Pierre reached out to him through their mutual friend Greg Jackson. "GSP contacted me through Greg Jackson. He gave me some advice and part of the message was how important the rehab was. You have to be careful and don't push it too hard, too fast. As athletes, we are risk takers, we want to push ourselves. But you need to be patient and trust the process. My advice for recovering from injuries is the same as my advice in general for reaching goals, and that is focusing on the small stuff — the day-to-day grind and task at hand, and to do well at that. Whether it's training for a fight or doing your therapy, it's the small incremental steps that get you to where you want to be. Having gone through ACL rehab, I took some exercises away from it, including working on stability. I spend a lot of time with my strength and conditioning coach on injury prevention exercises, mobility, and functional movement. It may be boring at times, but it prevents injury."

## THE IMPORTANCE OF MUSCULAR STABILITY

Some MMA athletes have actually been able to avoid surgery during their career by focusing on strengthening the large muscle groups around the knee and working on dynamic (active movement) stability such as plyometrics. If these muscle groups can prevent the athlete from experiencing the "giving way" feeling associated with a ruptured ACL, then reconstruction may not be necessary. Most surgeons, however, will argue that reconstructing the ACL will thwart further irreparable cartilage and meniscus damage. Furthermore, the athlete may not be able to perform at his peak if the knee isn't 100% stable. This is a significant discussion an athlete should have with his or her doctor.

Former UFC Light Heavyweight Champion Frank Shamrock avoided ACL reconstruction during his career, but not without some limitation: "My biggest knee injury was training for Phil Baroni in 2007 for an event co-promoted by Strikeforce and EliteXC. I was sparring a judo guy and he swept me and I couldn't walk for a week. The pain and swelling were severe. I tore my ACL. I saw three doctors and they all told me to do the rehab first and then do the surgery, so we could cut the rehab time in half. Rehab was challenging. At three months my knee was stable enough that I could fully train, so the doctor told me I had the option to avoid surgery."

Shamrock continues, "We focused heavily on balancing, building hamstrings, and loosening up the hip and calves so the knee stayed relaxed. It only bothered me during tennis. I fought about twice more without an ACL. However, it did affect my fighting. It affected my ability to shoot in and close the distance and also to step in and create power. I had to move forward at a more measured pace."

When it comes to putting your knees at risk, Frank points to shoes as one injury-causing issue during his career: "When I was in Pancrase, the shoe acted as a handle to lock your foot and hurt your knee. The same is true in wrestling when someone grabs your knee and you twist to get out. You can really hurt your knee. Do not let someone hang on your leg!"

Braces can support an injured knee, although sometimes they cannot withstand the forces generated by professional athletes during competition. There are many pictures out there that show a bent brace following a collision between NFL players. Braces come in several functional styles. The compression-sleeve braces help keep the knee warm and remind the athlete to focus on good form, but don't actually provide any mechanical stability. Hinged braces can help athletes recovering from ligament injuries feel more stable, but there is little evidence they do anything for actual injury prevention during competition. One study showed braces helped protect the MCL of football defensive players, but other than that, it seems they are more of a mental support for the athlete. Frank Shamrock would use his brace to keep his knee warm. However, the master of mind games that he is, he often would put it on the uninjured knee to distract his opponent's attention!

Ken Shamrock also had significant experience with ACL injuries during his long and impressive MMA career. "I tore my ACL while in Japan training for a fight, and Tra Telligman had to take the fight instead. He ended up getting an upset win over powerful Russian striker Igor Vovchanchyn at *Pride 13*," said Ken. "Afterwards, I had many fights with a torn ACL. It was actually torn during my first fight with Tito Ortiz. I had it fixed after that fight. We used a patella tendon graft. With a torn ACL, I felt I lost the ability to shoot and move on the ground for submissions. My training instead focused on stand-up. Once I had surgery, it was hard to get back to shooting, since I hadn't been doing it for so long. I had to retrain and rehab a lot to get deep knee bends for shooting in. I didn't do 100% of the rehab that I should have. Other sports don't need such deep knee bends that wrestling or grappling needs."

Shamrock goes on to say, "If you don't focus on those deep range of motion points, you may have a false sense of security. You may be able to do other activities or beat some guys, but it will take 12–15 months to get into those grappling positions you need to be in at the top of your game. You need to test your leg in all positions. Sit on your heels and try and lay back. Lunges are a great exercise to test the stability of the leg and strengthen the knee. These will help you find where you really are."

## MCL AND LCL INJURIES

On either side of the knee are the collateral ligaments: the MCL, medial (inner) collateral ligament, and LCL, lateral (outer) collateral ligament. These collateral ligaments are important in stabilizing the knee when a force is directed from either the inside or outside of the knee. If the knee is hit from the outside aspect of the knee, such as someone diving in for a tackle, the LCL compresses and the MCL stretches, making the MCL the important stabilizer of the knee at that moment. The opposite is true if the knee is hit from a force on the inner side of the knee and directed laterally; there, the LCL becomes tight and acts as the stabilizing ligament. The MCL and LCL can also be injured during grappling, when the knee is forced to bend at an awkward angle.

When the MCL is injured, it is usually sprained, in which some of the fibers stretch or break, but the ligament is not completely ruptured. This usually heals in a matter of weeks. If, however, the MCL completely ruptures, it can still heal on its own because it is enclosed in a sheath and can form a clot that allows reparative cells to lay down new tissue. It is for this reason the MCL rarely requires reparative surgery.

Pat Miletich suffered an MCL injury early in his career: "I was training for my first UFC four-man tournament [*UFC 16*]. I was up against the wall and my left leg was straight and locked. Two heavyweights were grappling by us and both guys landed on my left leg. I tore my MCL and had no insurance. I couldn't train. I could only jog on a treadmill. Three and a half months out, I couldn't bend my knee beyond 90 degrees.

"My wife, who was my girlfriend at the time, had been going to chiropractic college and knew some sports guys. We worked on stability drills and then iced my knee after the drills. A good exercise is to grab on to the side of a weight machine, push your foot down onto a swiss ball and do circular motions with your leg; one way 10 times and then 10 times the other way to build stability and proprioception. I also did leg raises sideways and at different angles while using an ankle weight. I went on to win the tournament."

When it comes to preventing these types of knee injuries, Pat feels flexibility is important: "It comes down to flexibility. Warm up [legs and knees] correctly, rotate them in circles, work on different angles. I learned this in wrestling. I was very flexible while in kickboxing. But then I didn't focus on flexibility in MMA. I was thinking I wouldn't need to kick high. That was a mistake. It certainly made me more prone to injuries during my career."

Two-time Strikeforce Lightweight Champion Gilbert Melendez has felt the pain of an MCL injury from being kicked on the outer part of the knee. The force caused the inner side of his knee to bend, injuring his MCL. "Everyone should learn how to properly block a kick. I have been kicked from the outside, which stretched my MCL. I was able tape it up, use a brace, and train through it. I could actually feel my knee wobble a little even when walking. It took about three to four weeks to heal. It's important to have a good tape job, which helps. Part of becoming a martial artist is evolving your game and learning new techniques. I was a boxer with a boxer's stance and have learned to train more Muay Thai. In Muay Thai, you turn your leg out to raise your knee and block your opponent's kick with your shin. It can hurt, but it's better than the kick hitting or stretching your ligaments. It can be simply lifting your knee and having good timing. But it takes practice. Also work on building the muscles around your knee. And watch how trainers properly tape hands, knees, and ankles. I enjoy taping my own joints and take my time doing it. To avoid injuries with kicking, don't aim for the knees. Aim for above the knee for both your safety and your partner's. Once, I asked my Muay Thai coach, 'When will it stop hurting to kick and block?' and he said, 'Never.' So I always wear pads and avoid hitting the joints with my kicks and blocks to minimize the risk of injury."

The LCL, however, is rarely injured in an isolated incident, although it can certainly happen in MMA. Usually the LCL is injured in a very high-impact injury, such as a car accident, and involves several other structures on the posterior and lateral side of the knee (a posterolateral injury), which can often involve the PCL. Again, like the MCL, it is more commonly sprained than completely ruptured and can usually heal on its own without surgery. However, surgery may be necessary if there is a multi-ligament injury involving the LCL/posterolateral corner and either the ACL or PCL, part of the LCL has pulled off with a fixable piece of bone, or when the knee is rotationally unstable.

## PCL INJURIES

Posterior Cruciate Ligaments (PCL) injuries are rare in sports, but are more common in mixed martial arts than in other sports. The PCL is usually injured when a significant force pushes the tibia backwards relative to the femur. In a motor vehicle accident, this may be referred to as a "dashboard injury" as a person hits the dashboard with their knee, driving the tibia backwards. In MMA, when a fighter shoots in towards an opponent, they often drive one or both of their own bent knees onto the mat, putting a backwards force onto the knee, stressing the PCL. Usually, the PCL is just sprained, but repeated sprains or one large force may result in a complete rupture of the PCL. If the PCL is completely ruptured, it may be reconstructed similar to an ACL, but usually it is treated with only rehabilitation, focusing on the quadriceps. Since the job of the PCL is to keep the tibia from moving backwards, strengthening the quadriceps can bring the tibia forward and help avoid PCL surgery. If a fighter continues to have instability despite proper rehabilitation, then a surgery can be offered. UFC heavyweight fighter and K-1 kickboxer Mark Hunt suffered a PCL injury during his fight with Jérôme Le Banner in the K-1 World Grand Prix but was able to avoid surgery for a long time. "It happened in front of eighty thousand people. It sounded like a crack from a whip!" recalls Hunt. "I started as a kick [boxing] fighter and have received more injuries in that sport than in MMA. When I was with K-1 it wasn't a matter of if you were going to be injured — it was a matter of how much. I actually started MMA because of the PCL injury. I was out for a year. When I came back, I had an offer from Pride. I had six weeks to train for my first fight, so I started doing jiu-jitsu."

Mark continues, "However, even after my PCL tore, I was still able to fight successfully for 10 more years without needing surgery. Then, when I was training with Antonio 'Bigfoot' Silva for my fight with Stefan Struve, he was kicking it, and I found out how bad my leg was. I went to my doctor and got an MRI. It was my PCL. He couldn't see anything left of it. Now, after surgery and proper rehab, the only lingering effect is I am not as fast moving with the left leg."

## MENISCUS INJURIES

One of the most overlooked, but perhaps most important, injuries related to a fighter's career is a meniscus injury. The meniscus acts as a shock distributor in the knee, but when it is torn, it can cause pain and result in other parts of the knee, such as the articular cartilage (joint cartilage on the bone), being damaged. Meniscus tears can be either simple or complex. If the meniscus tear is simple, it usually happened from a particular injury, as opposed to complex tears, which result from degeneration over time or repeated injury. Simple meniscus tears that occur in the outer third of the meniscus ring where the blood supply is best are candidates for repair with suture devices. All the other types of meniscus tears are usually shaved down to a smooth rim to prevent the torn flaps from catching within the knee and causing pain and mechanical locking.

UFC Welterweight Champion Matt Serra suffered a torn meniscus, but under the guidance of his doctor, he was able to avoid surgery and rehab his way back into the Octagon and to a historic title shot. "I tore my meniscus around 2006 while rolling jiu-jitsu. My ankle went in towards my chest and I felt a pain in my knee. I had torn my meniscus. Fortunately, my meniscus tear didn't need surgery. I worked on strengthening my knee and the muscles around it under the direction of my doctor and rehabbed it properly and got through it.

"Shortly after I got hurt, I got a call from the UFC for a fight against Karo Parisyan, who had just beaten Shonie Carter, Nick Diaz, and Chris Lytle. I took the fight, but had to train around my injury. I focused instead on my boxing skills, since my ability to roll was limited. In reality, the injury ended up being a blessing in disguise. By training around my injury, I improved my striking. I ended up losing to Karo, but that loss led me to *The Ultimate Fighter* (*TUF*) comeback show, which led to my title shot and KO victory over Georges St-Pierre."

Matt Serra's trainer, Ray Longo, recalls a similar story. "Matt hurt his meniscus, but it didn't need surgery. For the Karo Parisyan fight, we had to take out the jump squats and plyometric exercises that hurt his knee. It was also hard to work his cardio, so I worked on boxing and his exercises were done under the supervision of his doctor. When he lost, I made sure Matt never gave up. The most important thing was to keep Matt mentally in the game, even when he was dropped from the UFC. And then he got that call for *TUF: The Comeback*, and he seized the opportunity and never lost focus; and the rest, as they say, is history."

According to his trainer Mark DellaGrotte, Patrick Côté has battled many knee injuries, one of which sticks out in his mind. "In 2008, Côté had hurt his knee going into training camp against Anderson Silva. The bout was scheduled for the world title and Côté didn't want to pull out, so he continued training through the pain." In the process, Patrick had a cortisone shot to help with the pain and inflammation.

Sometimes a single cortisone shot can help an athlete get through a particular contest, but often the effects are only temporary, as the underlying injury is still there. Some doctors are also wary of repeated cortisone shots, as they can weaken tendons and ligaments and even lead to rupture of these structures.

**MARK DELLAGROTTE'S TOP THREE INJURIES HE SEES IN MMA TRAINING**

1. Knee Injuries
2. Hand Injuries
3. Skin Infections

Despite the pain, "The Predator" continued training for Anderson Silva. Côté didn't want to bail on a title fight with Silva. "Up to that point," Mark continues, "nobody had taken him past the second round and we wanted to put on a great fight. We had taken Silva into deep water where he had not been before. Côté was behind on the score cards, but we managed to take Silva, who was unstoppable at the time, all the way to the third round. Unfortunately, at the start of the third round, Côté's knee gave out and he dropped to the ground and was unable to continue. Patrick had maybe torn his meniscus even more, and the pain was severe enough that he required surgery. He ended up having a meniscus repair that kept him out of action afterwards for close to a year." This actually illustrates the dilemma a doctor and an athlete face between shaving or repairing a meniscus. If a meniscus tear is in the right location, it can be repaired in the hopes that it heals and preserves the meniscus. While waiting for the meniscus to heal (which it may not despite having surgery) the fighter will be out of action for several months. With a shaving, since you don't have to wait for a tear to heal, a fighter can get back quicker, but the shaving also takes away some of the meniscus in the process, limiting its effectiveness as a shock absorber and possibly increasing the risk of arthritis down the road.

Once a meniscus is damaged, it can no longer fully protect the articular cartilage of the knee. If the articular cartilage of the knee is damaged enough, early arthritis can set in and significantly limit a fighter's career. Since the meniscus is usually damaged with twisting injuries, it is important to keep the knee strong. In addition, untreated ACL injuries have been shown to set people up for meniscus injuries as well.

During the opening bout of the main card of *UFC on Fuel TV 5*, Duane "Bang" Ludwig, an MMA and Muay Thai veteran, collapsed with a knee injury. MRIs later revealed both a ruptured ACL and torn menisci. Duane's surgeon elected to repair the menisci and then schedule the ACL reconstruction after the meniscus repairs healed, because meniscus repairs often require the athlete to keep the knee from bending beyond 90 degrees until they heal. Other surgeons may do both surgeries at the same time since the blood in the knee released from the ACL drilling may actually help to heal the meniscus tear repair. Duane's surgery was done arthroscopically and his meniscus repair and torn ACL were documented.

Ken Shamrock has some advice for fighters who suffer meniscus and other soft-tissue injuries: "Guys need to understand these soft-tissue injuries may not seem like a big deal at the beginning, but in the long run they may see some serious side effects. Don't ignore your injuries and make sure to talk to the doctor about it. If not treated earlier on, you may end up tearing even more of your meniscus and having more surgeries and pretty soon the majority of it will be gone."

Dean Lister also has some advice on knee surgery for fighters. "Knee injuries were one of my big curses. If you need surgery, I suggest you just do it. In my case, I delayed surgery on my knee and ended up losing one year of my athletic career simply from denial. On the other hand, if you have an injury that doesn't need surgery, please don't be ashamed to practice on the sidelines. That will save your knee from further abuse until it is healed. And more importantly, be careful about the partners you select. A bad training partner can and will make things worse."

CSAC executive director Andy Foster echoes the importance of having good training partners for avoiding knee injuries. "As a former MMA fighter, I have injured my knees many times while grappling.

Make sure you are warmed up before engaging in grappling and/ or kickboxing. Also, when training heel hooks, toe holds, and knee bars, make sure that your partner knows to let go immediately and to not actually go for the tap. That's a key difference. A good training partner with a safe training plan will greatly eliminate knee injuries associated with grappling. Sometimes knee injuries occur when practicing takedowns. I would suggest only practicing takedowns in a wrestling room with qualified trainers. A blown knee can damage a promising combat-sports career. I suggest wearing good equipment and even wrapping your knees for support. In Muay Thai, make sure your partner is trustworthy and does not target the knee or the kneecap. Also be careful with 'axe-kicks,' as I have seen ligament hyperextension injuries from these getting blocked. Finally, this is more than obvious but it is worth pointing out: do not spar hard with people you do not know."

## QUADRICEPS AND PATELLAR TENDON INJURIES

At the top of the knee, the quadriceps muscles thicken and condense to form the quadriceps tendon. This tendon can be partially or completely ruptured. Complete ruptures require surgery, but partial ruptures can be healed through proper rehab. In his preparation for *UFC Fight For the Troops 3*, army veteran Tim Kennedy suffered a partial tear of his quadriceps tendon. "During fight camp, your body fat is low. You are like a thoroughbred horse. You are trained exactly to do what you need to fight three or five 5-minute rounds. I was finishing up my 10-week fight camp and was doing my last strength and conditioning session. My body was at 4% body fat, and I am normally around 8%. I was out on the track running hard, and a lady walked over the track. It was either run over a 65-year-old lady and probably kill her, or try to decelerate in about two meters. I chose to decelerate and just fell to the ground, grabbing my leg and screaming. I partially tore my quadriceps, but I knew I had to fight for the troops. Fortunately, I knocked my opponent out in the first round. I didn't suffer any further injuries and went straight into rehabbing my knee. First, I rested for two weeks after my fight. Then I began working on linear and lateral movements. I worked on building back up the muscle atrophy with electrical stimulation. I used deep tissue massage. Then I began formal physical therapy."

As the quadriceps run over the top of the femur, they insert onto the patella (knee cap). The patella is then connected to the tibia by the patellar tendon. The patellar tendon can be partially or completely ruptured or it can become inflamed by repetitive stress. This inflammation of the patellar tendon is called patellar tendonitis. Repetitive jumping or kicking can lead to patellar tendonitis. If the patellar tendon does become inflamed, it can be treated with rest and anti-inflammatories. Some fighters may find a small strap that goes over the end of the tendon to be helpful. If the patellar tendon is completely ruptured, it will need to be surgically repaired.

Tendonitis tends to come from overuse, which may happen later in a fighter's career. In addition to anti-inflammatories, some doctors may offer a cortisone shot. In his experience, Cesar Gracie's fighters tend to seek out a cortisone injection when they have an upcoming fight they can't, or won't, pull out of. "Tendonitis generally comes in the second part of a guy's career. There is a lot of pressure for a guy to perform. He has to be ready to go. If he doesn't fight, he doesn't get paid and his trainer doesn't get paid. You may lose your spot in the line to the big fight. Sometimes a cortisone shot is what it takes." If you are considering a cortisone shot, talk to your doctor and be sure you aren't using cortisone too much. It's a temporary solution, so make sure to address whatever the underlying problem is.

Another option under active investigation for tendonitis and partial tendon tears throughout the body is the use of platelet-rich plasma (PRP). With PRP, a small amount of blood is taken from the patient and spun in a centrifuge to separate out the cells from the healing factors and signaling molecules normally circulating in the body's blood. With the centrifuge, these factors are concentrated down into a small vial, which can then be injected directly into the site of injury in hopes of reducing inflammation and promoting healing. The exact method of healing isn't fully known and each company's preparation is a little different, so talk to your doctor about his or her experience with PRP and what the cost to you would be, as it's not usually covered by insurance.

## INJURY PREVENTION

The key to preventing injury to knee ligaments and the meniscus is proper biomechanics of the knee joint. Strengthening the large muscle groups around the knee joint such as the quadriceps and hamstring muscles helps to keep the knee properly aligned when the muscles contract. Exercises such as leg extensions and hamstring curls, which isolate each muscle group, are important for building strength. However, these exercises alone are often not enough to help prevent injury in a dynamic sport.

Improving neuromuscular control is critical for the moments when a fighter suddenly slips, gets tripped, or twists a leg during grappling. The body has a neuromuscular network that works on a subconscious level, similar to our reaction to pulling our hand off a hot stove. We don't think about it, our muscles just contract and we do it. The same can be applied to knee injuries. If the knee is suddenly tweaked, the large muscle groups may contract quickly to help stabilize it. However, it's important that the muscles contract in the appropriate sequence. Exercises that help this happen are more dynamic and plyometric exercises such as box jumps, single-leg squats and hops, and shuttle runs. In addition, especially for women, working on proper hip, knee, and foot alignment and positioning while landing from jumps has been shown to prevent ligament injuries.

Besides proper mechanics, a good training environment can help prevent the unexpected knee injury. Well-known striking coach Mike Winkeljohn points out some things he and Greg Jackson have learned while training some of UFC's top fighters. "Some injuries are just unavoidable. Jon Jones's knee injury was unavoidable. When Jon hurt his knee, our problem was not enough space. It's not the one-on-one encounters that hurt most guys in our camp, it's being blindsided by someone or something. Often our gym gets crowded because everyone wants to be there at the same time, and this can lead to guys rolling into each other and causing injuries. It sounds simple, but it's important. Also, if mats are too sticky or too spongy, you can't rotate your grounded foot with your kick or during takedown. That can lead to a lot of torque on your knee. When kicking, such as with a roundhouse, don't push into the ground. Your ground foot should be hovering ever so slightly. Turn your foot before you kick or rotate with the kick. Send all your force into your opponent, not into the ground."

UFC Heavyweight and Lightweight Champion Randy Couture echoes this statement, especially during transition drills from standing to grappling. "For takedown and transition drills, watch out for wet or sweaty mat surfaces, overcrowded spaces, and cracks or crevices in flooring. Those can be major causes of injuries with those drills." Jiu-jitsu world champion and American Top Team (ATT) co-founder Ricardo Liborio thinks the type of mats used can limit injuries. "In Brazil, where we do mostly grappling, the mats are more like the puzzle mats. But here at ATT, for MMA we use the rolling mats since there are less places to get caught. I have seen it often, if the puzzle mats get out of place and a hole opens up you can get your hand or leg caught, especially in wrestling or when you start standing up for MMA and takedowns. Plus, the rolling mats are easier to clean."

Perhaps the easiest piece of advice for knee and overall injury prevention comes from UFC Welterweight Champion Carlos Newton. "The closest thing to a significant knee injury I have had was when I was younger and doing Brazilian Jiu-Jitsu. My partner was a sambo practitioner and while I was in sidemount, he decided to grab my leg in a knee bar and pull my leg sideways — it left me very tender. I learned in that instant, I wanted to avoid injuries while grappling, to not get knee barred and not to fight a submission attempt while you're rolling. When grappling, it is important to not let your ego rule. I was able to avoid injury by not pushing through moves in wrestling, judo, and BJJ. Judo is notorious for knee injuries, but you can develop the skill of avoiding risky positions. Not getting injured is actually a skill in itself, and I made sure to develop it. That same skill actually helps avoid opportunities for my opponents to attack. Certain angles of attack and certain positions put you at risk for injury and give your opponents an attacking advantage."

Greg Nelson, a former NCAA wrestler and the coach of top MMA wrestlers and champions Sean Sherk and Brock Lesnar, sees two things as leading to knee injury during grappling. The first is not knowing the proper technique or reversal of a knee bar, heel hook, or similar move, and the other is an aggressive grappler who attempts to explode out of a bad position. "Knee injuries are pretty common and can happen in both training and fights. Due to the nature of MMA and the intensity of the scrambles, takedowns, and guards, it is easy for a fighter to tweak their knee. Like wrestling, a lot of knee injuries happen when a fighter attempts to win a scramble and fight for top position. I can recount a number of occasions when a fighter had their foot get caught on the mat at a funny angle or their opponent had a hold of it while they quickly jerked their body away. The twisting, combined with quick, jerky movements makes for easy knee tweaks, sprains, or torn cartilage/ligaments. Many of these injuries stem from making an explosive motion without really knowing where they are going to end up. In other words, there is no planned technical response, just a reactionary explosive movement. This is more likely to happen with a very intense individual that is always attempting to be more explosive than technical.

"Leg locks are also a major cause of knee injuries, especially the reverse heel hook. Injuries occur during leg locks when either (1) the attacker quickly hits the lock, be it a heel hook or straight knee bar, and doesn't give his partner sufficient time to tap, or (2) the fighter who is getting leg locked explosively attempts to get away and in the process damages their own knee. It is crucial during training that those grappling live understand that leg locks directly torque the knee, and they must learn to control their pressure when applying the lock. It's also vital to learn proper escape techniques and know when to tap when caught. I do not allow new students to do twisting leg locks or knee bars (only Achilles locks and straight ankle locks), making sure they first learn how to properly counter and know when to tap. This is hard when you have two very competitive fighters who are proficient at leg locks."

Nelson goes on to talk about another area of concern, which happens when an aggressive wrestler-type is relentless in passing the guard. In this scenario, the bottom fighter refuses to open his guard and allows his legs to get into an odd angle, and then the top fighter, in an aggressive and explosive manner, throws his opponent's legs and drops his weight down onto the bottom opponent. During this type of scenario if the top partner drops quickly and the bottom is not ready . . . POP! There goes the knee. My instructor, Professor Pedro Sauer, told me never to put your knees in a position that, if the top person were to drop all their weight down suddenly, your knees would not be able to bend naturally."

During the height of his career, Sean Sherk often overlooked injury prevention, and he suffered the consequences. "Based on my experience, guys don't do any preventative exercises until it's too late. I trained pretty hard. If something didn't hurt, I wouldn't worry about it. Once something hurt, I would just work through it. If it got to the point where I couldn't work through it on a regular basis, I would throw a brace on it. Eventually it would be 'done' and I would need surgery."

Having suffered a knee injury before and having had to work to get back from surgery, Tim Kennedy knows the importance of focusing on injury prevention. "I spend about 90 minutes for a training session. Two-thirds of that is dedicated to injury prevention, mostly core and muscle stretching and strengthening. Also doing band work and [working with] training balls. Olympic lifts and sprints are only about one-third of my workout. The vast majority is injury prevention."

# KNEE INJURY PREVENTION EXERCISES

Part of knee injury prevention is maintaining good balance and core strength, while good biomechanics help to keep the hips and knees aligned, avoiding stress on the ligaments. Below are some dynamic control and core strengthening/balance exercises that can help fortify the muscles around the knee and prevent knee injuries.

To work on core strength and balance, you can hold a medicine ball while standing on one foot and rotate to either side.

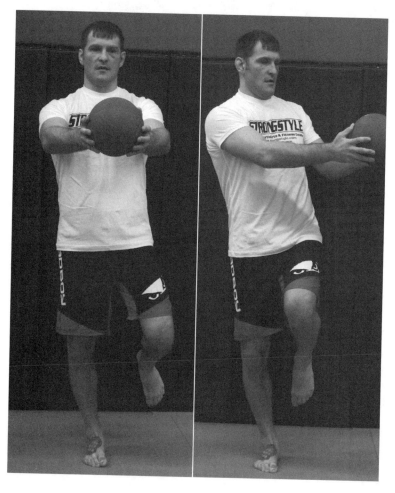

Repeat using a lunge position.

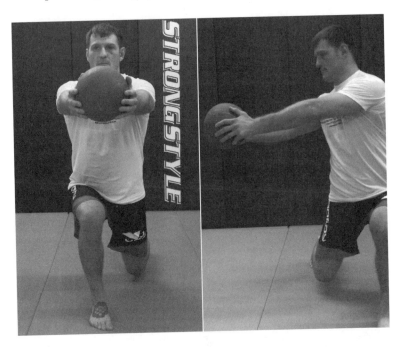

Have a partner throw the ball to you so you can catch it on one leg, rotate, and throw it back.

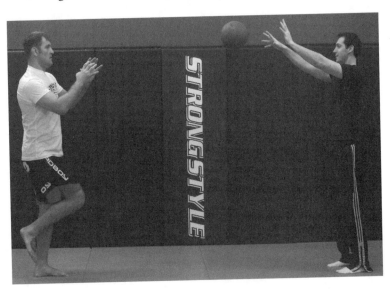

Lunges and one-legged squats help keep muscles strong but also help teach the body to keep appropriate alignment. To avoid injury, remember not to bend your knees past 90 degrees. You can also look at your knee from above and make sure you can still see your toes to make sure you haven't bent your knees too much.

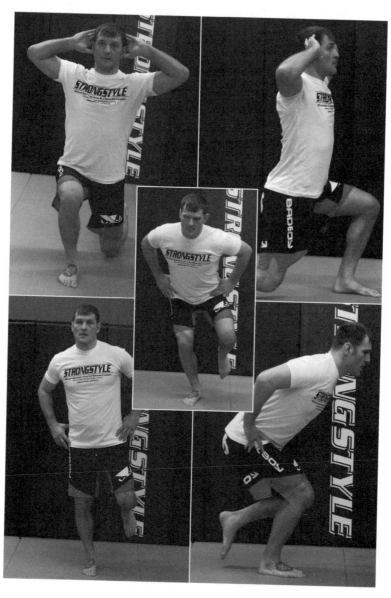

Resistance bands can be placed around the legs for lateral shuffling. Make sure your knees and hips are pointing outward and not inward, which stress the knee ligaments.

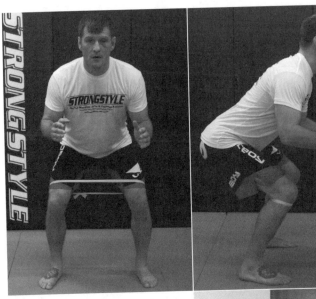

Plyometrics and rapid sequence movements help train the body to function in appropriate positions and maintain good form at a rapid pace. These can include box jumps,

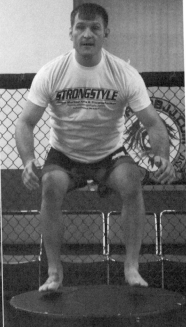

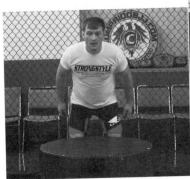

lateral one-legged landings,

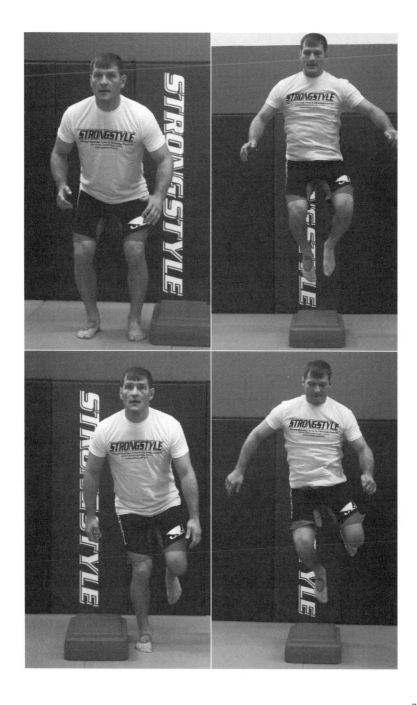

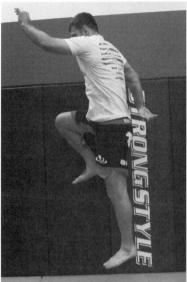

◄ high-stepping,

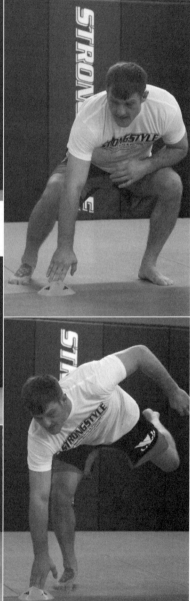

lateral shuttle runs, ►

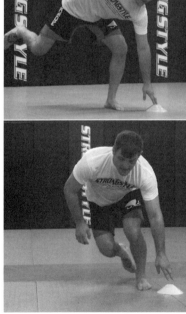

and running drills where you and your partner cross over each other.

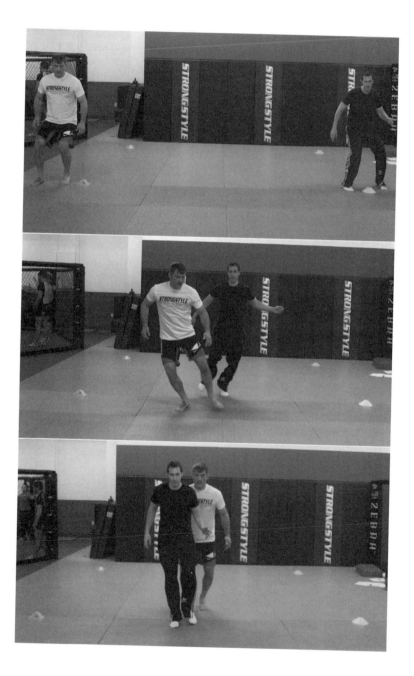

Traditional exercises such as leg press, leg extension, wall squats, and leg curls help to isolate muscle groups. The leg extension and leg curls are called "open-chain" exercises, because they isolate either the quadriceps or hamstring muscle groups.

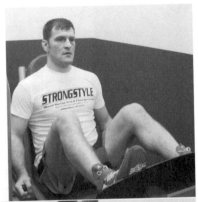

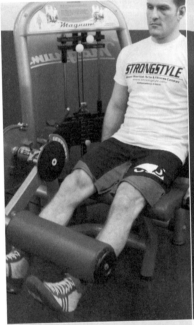

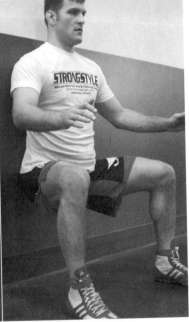

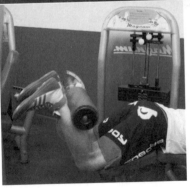

The leg press and wall squats are called "closed-chain" exercises because they activate both muscle groups together.

## CHAPTER 5

# SHOULDER INJURIES AND HOW AN INJECTION CHANGED THE ODDS IN VEGAS

Strikeforce Lightweight Champion Gilbert Melendez still bears the deformity of his 2012 shoulder injury. "Gilbert was in one of his final all-out practices, grappling with his teammate Jake Shields," states his father and manager Gilbert Melendez Sr. "Jake is much bigger than my son, and they were battling on a takedown and neither man wanted to give it up. They fell to the mat and Gilbert landed hard on his shoulder and ended up separating it." The bump from the separated acromioclavicular joint is still apparent after his injury, so much so that UFC commentator Joe Rogan commented on Gilbert's "funky" shoulder six months later during his UFC bout against Benson Henderson.

Since it mainly depends on how you land, throws are where a lot of shoulder injuries happen. According to well-known trainer Mark DellaGrotte, "Judo throws don't allow you to land as safely as a wrestling-style takedown. As opposed to a single- or double-leg takedown, with a judo throw you go head over heels and are often disoriented and don't know where the mat is and can't break your fall. This results in a lot of guys landing on their head or injuring their shoulders. I train a lot of judo black-belts and Olympians, so I have seen a lot of this firsthand."

## ANATOMY

After the knee, the shoulder is probably the most commonly injured, and discussed, joint. The shoulder provides a huge range of motion, but it does so by sacrificing some stability. In essence, the shoulder is made up of a ball-and-socket joint, similar to a large golf ball on a small tee. The ball of the shoulder is the head, or top part, of the humerus (arm bone). It sits in a shallow cup of the shoulder blade called the glenoid. The edge of the glenoid is deepened by the labrum (a ring of cartilage), which acts as a bumper and stabilizes the head in the socket. The shoulder blade also has a bony projection called the acromion that comes up and around to meet the clavicle (collar-bone). This is called the acromioclavicular (AC) joint.

The ball of the shoulder joint is held in place by ligaments, the labrum, and the pull of the rotator cuff muscles.

In addition to the ligaments and rotator cuff, the large muscle groups around the shoulder such as the deltoid, latissimus dorsi, and

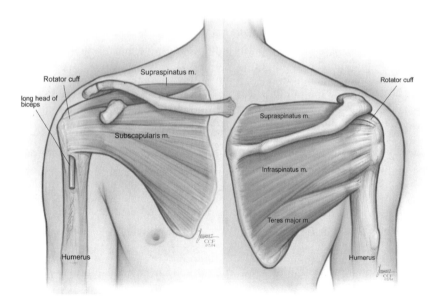

FRONT AND BACK VIEWS OF THE SHOULDER, SHOWING THE ROTATOR CUFF, LONG HEAD OF THE BICEPS, AND ACROMIOCLAVICULAR JOINT.
CREDIT: JOE KANASZ.

trapezius help keep the shoulder in alignment and take some of the stress off of the rotator cuff and shoulder ligaments.

## SHOULDER DISLOCATIONS

The most dramatic shoulder injury is a dislocation (not to be confused with an AC separation, which is discussed later). In a shoulder dislocation, the ball dislocates completely from the socket, which is what happened to MMA veteran Josh Barnett. While working for position on the ground during the beginning of the first round at *Pride 28*, Barnett suddenly tapped, ending the fight. "I dislocated my shoulder 30 seconds into my first fight with Mirko "Cro Cop" [Filipovic]. I had torn my labrum in training, and then during the fight, I got put into a bad position with a takedown. I couldn't do anything about it — my shoulder was unstable. I needed surgery. I was out for eight months and my left shoulder will never have as much mobility as my right. My advice is to strengthen your shoulder and your rotator cuff muscles. If you do work the small muscles like the rotator cuff, don't use a lot of weight. Work on stability exercises and isometric holds. Work on mobility, but not hypermobility. Whether it's a shoulder, elbow, or knee, don't take things to extreme mobility and don't hammer your joints."

The shoulder can dislocate anteriorly (forwards) or posteriorly (backwards). The vast majority of shoulder dislocations are anterior, as the arm is usually pulled away from the body driving the ball forward. As the ball moves out of the socket, it can tear a piece of the labrum or break off a piece of bone from the socket. If this happens, it can lead to chronic shoulder instability and multiple dislocations. Surgery can help prevent this by repairing the torn labrum or bone, but it is up to the fighter and his doctor as to whether they should repair it right away or wait to see if there are more dislocations. Treating a shoulder dislocation with surgery will likely prevent repeated visits to the emergency room, but it will also put the fighter on the shelf for a while as they heal.

If a shoulder does become dislocated during training or a match, a fighter or his camp may try to put it back in themselves. However,

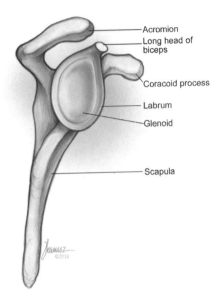

- Acromion
- Long head of biceps
- Coracoid process
- Labrum
- Glenoid
- Scapula

VIEW OF THE GLENOID SOCKET IN THE SCAPULA WITH THE BICEPS ATTACHING AT THE TOP OF THE GLENOID INSIDE THE SHOULDER.
CREDIT: JOE KANASZ.

this can sometimes cause further injury — including broken bones. If this happens during training and there are no doctors or certified athletic trainers around, the best thing to do is go to the emergency room. If the dislocation only happened a little while before the visit, it usually can be put back into place without difficulty. If a dislocation happens at an event, the ringside physician may elect to reduce the dislocation in the locker room or transport the fighter to the hospital for better medication. Either way, if a simple shoulder dislocation is reduced, the fighter can wear a sling for a few days for comfort, but in most cases it's best to start a comfortable and gentle range of motion as soon as possible to prevent the shoulder from getting stiff.

## AC SEPARATIONS

An injury that is often confused with a shoulder dislocation is an AC sprain, also referred to as an AC separation. The AC stands for acromioclavicular, which means it is a joint formed between the acromion, which comes up and over the top of the shoulder blade, and the clavicle. When a fighter lands on their shoulder, they can cause this joint to separate, leading to an AC separation. The level of separation is graded based on how much the bones separate from each other. Lower grades are usually just sprains and can be treated with a sling until the pain gets better and the fighter gradually returns to training. The treatment of some higher grades, especially a grade

III where all ligaments are torn and the clavicle is completely dislocated from the acromion, can be controversial. Some doctors will repair these with surgery, others will allow them to heal on their own. Surgery is done to prevent instability of the joint and, theoretically, to help with biomechanics. Without surgery, the joint can often heal with minimal limitations, but the fighter will have a permanent bump similar to Gilbert Melendez.

Melendez recalls how bad the injury initially looked, but also how quickly he was able to recover once the pain started to go away. "Jake went for an arm toss, and lot of times you can roll through it, but instead I resisted. I suddenly felt a lot of pain. The looks on my teammates' faces were pretty bad at the time. But at about three weeks from my injury, I started doing some light training and hitting pads. It took about eight to 10 weeks before I could fully use my shoulder. I actually ended up separating it again, but I didn't even notice. It looks weird, but it only minimally affects me."

## ROTATOR CUFF TEARS AND TENDONITIS

The rotator cuff, which helps hold the ball of the shoulder joint in place in its socket, is made up of four muscles: the supraspinatus, infraspinatus, teres minor, and subscapularis. Injuries to the rotator cuff fall on a spectrum from tendonitis (inflammation of the tendon) to partial and complete tears of one or more tendons. Usually when an athlete has a tear in the rotator cuff, it mostly involves the supraspinatus.

Partial tears of the rotator cuff present a challenge for the fighter and his doctor, as the pain from partial tears can either improve with rest and therapy or the tears may progress to full thickness, which can mean surgery and time off from fighting. Therefore, partial tears can initially be treated similarly to tendonitis with rest, anti-inflammatories, and proper therapy. UFC Welterweight Champion Pat Miletich suffered a rotator cuff injury during training. "I got thrown head first into the mat and threw my arm out and kicked my feet out to stop myself. The mat was completely covered in sweat. My arm flew behind my body and the guy let go of me right away, but I couldn't use my arm for eight months. I used water-resistance training a lot to rebuild it. I also focused on rotator cuff raises and using my hand as a paddle under water. Once I could lift my arm up again, I would start telescoping my fist into swiss balls at different angles. I still do the exercises to maintain strength of the muscles around the joint and protect my shoulder. I also like to swim laps."

However, if the tear is significant enough, the fighter is losing strength, and the pain is not improving, then surgery may be the solution. The surgery may be done through a small open incision or arthroscopically with the use of cameras and small instruments. In either case, the tendon is tacked back down to where it was torn off. However, if the injury is old, the muscle/tendon can become weaker, fattier, and retract so much so that the repair may not hold. That is why it is important to see a doctor for an exam and possibly an MRI as soon as you suspect a rotator cuff tear. And if you do have surgery, do not smoke cigarettes. The nicotine in the cigarettes causes the blood vessels to constrict, thereby reducing the bloodflow your tendon needs to heal.

Sean Sherk's trainer and coach Greg Nelson recalls how an incident involving Sean's shoulder actually affected the fight odds in Las Vegas one night before the event. "Sean had a great training camp leading up to his championship fight with Kenny Florian. We were coming up with new and creative drills to improve his guard passing and top control, while at the same time continuing to improve his lightning-fast shot. Ten days before the fight, Sean shot in for a double on one of our bigger fighters. Mistake number one was working with a bigger fighter with a great sprawl. Sean had shot in and his teammate sprawled and dropped his weight perfectly on Sean's shoulder. In a split second, Sean went from 100% healthy to having a torn rotator cuff and a grade II AC separation. He continued to train but could not use that arm with any real strength. Considering he was fighting for the 155 pound UFC lightweight title, not fighting was not an option.

"Sean met with a doctor and told him he wanted to fight, so what could he do to decrease the pain and give him a better range of motion? The doctor gave him a cortisone injection to relieve the inflammation, giving him increased range of motion and decreased pain." [Doctor's note: While cortisone injections can reduce inflammation acutely, repeated injections are controversial due to the risk of complications, including nerve damage, joint infections, cartilage damage, and tendon weakness.]

Nelson continues, "Later, the doctor at the UFC event asked Sean, in front of Kenny, which shoulder he got an injection in. Sean immediately said, 'It was my knee.' The doctor, looking at his papers said, "No, this said you had a cortisone injection in your shoulder." Up until that point we had kept the shoulder injury away from everyone. Prior to the doctor saying that in front of Kenny, and who knows who else heard, Sean was a 3 to 1 favorite to win. Within an hour after the pre-fight medical exam, the odds in Las Vegas went to even. Regardless, Sean ran through Kenny's guard and dominated the fight, beating Kenny Florian by unanimous decision to win the UFC lightweight title belt."

Winning the belt, however, is not the end of Sean's story on rotator cuff injuries. "When I tore my rotator cuff 10 days before fighting for the UFC championship, it was hard to make a decision whether or not to fight. I couldn't sleep or train, but I still made it to the fight and won the championship. I then had the surgery one week after the fight, but quickly tore it again. A big issue was that I just didn't take enough time to properly rehab. I trained too hard too soon." With surgery, the end of the story does not occur when you wake up in the recovery room after an operation. It continues long after with proper rehab and physical therapy. Even with partial, non-operative tears, rehab is important, and understanding the anatomy of the shoulder is the first step in setting up a proper recovery program.

Like partial and full tears, rotator cuff tendonitis is also very painful, especially with overhead activities. The first treatment for tendonitis is to take anti-inflammatories and rest from activities that aggravate the shoulder. Once the pain subsides, the fighter should focus on proper biomechanics to make sure the shoulder is moving smoothly, as well as to strengthen the large muscle groups around the shoulder to take some of the stress off the rotator cuff.

## BICEPS TENDONITIS

The biceps has two heads. One tendon is attached to the coracoid, a bone below the clavicle. The other tendon actually goes across the top of the shoulder joint and attaches to the top of the socket. The part of the biceps that runs inside the shoulder joint can become inflamed and irritated, leading to biceps tendonitis, which feels like pain in the front of the shoulder. Pain in this location can greatly hinder a fighter's training. This is exactly what happened to MMA legend Bas Rutten.

The former UFC Heavyweight Champion and three-time King of Pancrase World Champion had multiple bouts of biceps tendonitis throughout his career. "I would say my knees and tendonitis that I have in both arms are my biggest injuries. When I hit a bag too hard, or I have to use a lot of power to defend an arm submission, then there was always the chance the tendonitis would start, and when it did, training would be a nightmare every day — very painful."

For Bas, rest was the best treatment for his biceps tendonitis, but as a professional athlete he couldn't stop training, so he would work around the injury. "The doctor would say, 'No training,' but of course that wasn't a possibility. I would train around the arm — sometimes arms — and just kick and do sprinting drills. I tried ultrasound, laser, anything they had out there. Rest would be the best. That's my line to my students."

## BICEPS RUPTURES FROM THE SHOULDER

The long head of the biceps inside the shoulder can actually rupture or be purposefully cut and reattached by a surgeon to relieve shoulder pain. While training for an upcoming fight, UFC Welterweight Champion Carlos Newton felt an odd sensation in his shoulder. "I was sparring inside the cage. I had a move I often did when someone went for a double-leg takedown; I would do a high crotch counter, pick him up with one arm, and flip him on his back. One day, my partner shot in, I did a side step, countered, and lifted with one arm, and he went straight up in the air like I was going to throw him out of the cage. At that moment, I felt something snap softly in my shoulder. Everyone looked at me, and there was a little divot at the top of my shoulder by the biceps. I sat out a few minutes, and then returned to training for a little bit, but something felt wrong. So I called it a day and went to see my doctor. It looked to him like a partially torn biceps. I had an MRI, and the next day he said it was a partial tear, which they normally don't do anything for. I suggested getting the opinion of a surgeon. I wanted to keep training and wanted to make sure I didn't put my biceps at risk for further injury. After examining me and my MRI, the surgeon suggested going in and looking with a shoulder arthroscopy in three weeks' time.

"I had the go ahead to train in the meantime, so I kept training and had a great three weeks of training right up until the day of surgery. The surgeon went in and saw that the biceps was completely torn off the insertion into the shoulder. It had been completely torn but never slid down, so it looked only like a partial tear on the MRI. Since it was completely torn, he reinserted it into my arm bone through a small hole. I was back to training in about six weeks with no loss of motion, strength, or discomfort." What Carlos describes is called a biceps tenodesis — reattaching the biceps into the arm bone. Some athletes have had the long head of the biceps tear in the shoulder and actually felt pain relief from the tear, and they continued to play without any issues. John Elway actually won two Super Bowls without ever having surgery after his biceps ruptured from its attachment in the shoulder of his throwing arm.

## BICEPS RUPTURES AT THE ELBOW

As mentioned, the muscle of the biceps starts at the shoulder and ends by inserting at the elbow. It is at this insertion where athletes can also rupture their biceps. Contrary to popular belief, the biceps is not the main flexor of the elbow — that's the brachialis muscle. Matt Serra tore his biceps, and both he and his trainer, Ray Longo, feel it commonly occurs when guys are dehydrated, tight, and tired. Matt remembers, "I was training for *UFC 36* against Kelly Dullanty. I wasn't used to cutting weight the right way and I was dehydrated. I was sparring and I got lit up by a Golden Glover. During the sparring session, I tore my biceps. I did lose some strength, but I managed to win the fight with my legs by triangle choke."

Ray Longo adds, "I saw Matt throw an overhead punch, and right away, I could see it rolled up into his shoulder. We had a decision to make. Do you fight? Do you have surgery? He wanted to avoid surgery and fight. He had a deformity but only lost a little strength. He had 10 fights since the injury. He has a deformity, but he has done well. Back then, we fought with injuries, but now the stakes are a little higher and the careers can be more lucrative. My job as a coach is safety first and getting a guy to the fight as healthy as possible.

"If you hurt your arm or your shoulder, you have to keep moving. Don't just give up and sit on the couch. Talk your doctor and see what you can do. We can work around it. I had a kickboxer who had the same injury and had it surgically repaired and did well. The biggest risk, to me, is dehydration. As they get close to the fight, the fighters are dehydrated and tired. When you are training, you need to stay hydrated and get lots of sleep. As a coach, you need stay on top of the athletes to stay hydrated and rest up so their body has a chance to recover and heal."

## LABRAL TEARS/SLAP LESIONS

The labrum is the rim of cartilage that runs around the shoulder socket to help deepen it and provide additional stability. If a shoulder dislocates, the labrum can be torn, causing the ball to continue to dislocate. If the labrum tears at the top, it may be referred to as a SLAP lesion, which stands for superior (up top) labrum, torn anterior to posterior (from front to back). This particular injury may occur when the arm is severely rotated backwards or jarred directly upwards.

Where the SLAP lesions occur on the labrum is also where the biceps attaches inside the shoulder joint. The treatment for a SLAP tear depends on a fighter's symptoms. He or she may be able to rest it and train without pain afterwards. However, if surgery is needed, the torn labrum and biceps can be tacked back down to the shoulder socket. Sometimes the biceps tendon needs to be cut and reattached farther down the arm. The recovery may take several months and the results of SLAP repairs are not as promising in people over the age of 40. The best way to diagnose this injury is by a physical examination and MRI.

Before *UFC 172*, Brazilian Glover Teixeira was in a 20-fight win streak over seven years. At the same time, UFC Light Heavyweight Champion Jon Jones was on a streak of his own, 10 wins including six successful title defenses. Glover was known for his heart and his fortitude, but many fighters have never been the same after facing the champion, and Glover was added to that list. American Top Team coach Ricardo Liborio recalls when Glover injured his labrum. "John Hackleman and I were in Glover's corner. In the first round, Jones applied a standing arm-bar and shoulder crank. When Glover came back between rounds, his shoulder was huge and swollen, twice as big as the other one. He didn't complain, but just asked for some ice. So, we put one bag of ice on his neck and another on his shoulder. He fought the rest of the match, ultimately losing to Jon Jones via unanimous decision. An MRI later revealed he had torn his labrum, but fortunately was able to avoid surgery."

UFC Heavyweight Champion Cain Velasquez has actually suffered two torn labrums, one in each arm. His head coach at AKA, Javier Mendez, recalls the injuries: "Cain suffered labral tears in 2010 and 2013. The first one, in 2010, was against Brock Lesnar, and the other was in 2013 in his third fight against Junior dos Santos. Both needed surgery. When the JDS fight was over, Cain basically told me, 'I think I hurt my shoulder again.' After he cooled down, he was still hurting, so we went to get an MRI. There was a slight tear and he tried to rehab it for a few weeks but ended up needing surgery."

The first-ever UFC Flyweight Champion Demetrious Johnson also tore his labrum and required surgery. He remembers, "It hurt even brushing my teeth. I had arthroscopic debridement and PRP [platelet-rich plasma] injections. I rehabbed for six weeks, working on range of motion and flexibility. I did some reverse grip pull-ups. Swimming is also good. To prevent it [from happening] again, I keep my deltoid, latissimus, and pectoral muscles strong. I also stay away from heavier guys during training."

As with any injury, rehab time is vital, and Javier Mendez makes sure all his fighters get the proper clearance before they can return to the Octagon: "We follow the doctors' and therapists' advice exactly as they tell us. As a head coach and trainer, I have to enforce this. Sometimes, with a guy who really wants to get back too soon, the only thing I can do is lock them out of the gym. I know how fighters are and I want to hear it directly from the doctor. Even with Cain. I trust Cain, but when he said the doctor cleared him for light striking, I contacted the doctor directly to get clearance."

## GOING SLOW WITH SHOULDER REHAB

Frank Shamrock describes his encounter with a SLAP tear, "I had a SLAP tear in my right shoulder from throwing a punch. I was training with a boxer using 16 oz gloves, got him in a corner, and tried to punch him in the head, missed him, and felt the pain immediately. I fought two weeks later in the K-1 World Grand Prix against Elvis Sinosic and won by split decision. Later, I had arthroscopic surgery to fix it. After I recovered, I felt better and could achieve a full range of motion."

Frank then goes on to explain his rehabilitation program for this injury, "For shoulder therapy, using the shaking bow was useful. It made a huge difference for me. Also, walking forward or back with the swiss ball under me and using the swiss ball to 'write' letters with my hand. I also focused on stretching and relaxing the muscles of my upper body. I noticed I often tensed up too much when I threw a punch, and that may have contributed to why I tore it.

"Shoulder injury prevention is all about keeping loose and flexible. You need to keep them strong with a structured regimen. All of my workouts begin with assessing flexibility and then warming up. I end all of my workouts with a review to see what feels tight and focus on achieving a good relaxation and range of motion. Using my arms in water helped keep my shoulder and arms strong and flexible. I would just get in the water and move them."

It takes an extensive amount of time and effort to recover from a shoulder injury, which is why it's one of the most feared injuries in MMA. Since the pain will force you to take time off from moving the shoulder, it's likely that atrophy of the arm muscles will occur. This means taking the time to rehab is necessary to keep your strength and range of motion. As Cesar Gracie warns, "Shoulder injuries affect everything. Your arm, your chest, your back all hurt. With a shoulder injury, you are limited in MMA fighting." MMA champion and elite grappler Dean Lister has also had experiences with shoulder injuries, rehab, and prevention. He understands the importance of seeing qualified doctors to evaluate these joints before it's too late, and he agrees that shoulders tend to take a long time to heal. "Shoulder injuries are extremely complex. Many athletes such as myself have torn both shoulders badly. This is why some fighters cannot perform simple daily activities. I know some fighters that still fight but cannot lift up their own children. The shoulders are a complicated area — so pay a lot of attention to them. There are several rotator cuff warm-ups you can employ for training that will help with your athletic future. If you do have a serious shoulder injury that does require surgery, stick with your rehab in a steady manner. It can be frustrating, but in my experience shoulders tend to heal slower than other injuries, so don't jeopardize your recovery by going too fast too soon."

Much of recovering from an injury is understanding your body and focusing on other ways to improve. It's hard for a fighter to stop training completely, so being smart about what parts of your body you exercise can allow you to recover from an injury, while continuing to train. To Gilbert Melendez, "Recovering or working around an injury is mental. When I hurt my shoulder, I had to say to myself, I can use my legs and run. I can use my other hand. There are so many aspects to MMA that can keep you busy. I started experimenting with light resistance therapy bands and focus on my body awareness. Strong body awareness comes with slow movements and stretching."

The shoulder is a naturally unstable joint. The ball just barely fits into the cup. In order to keep it healthy, it's important to keep the large muscle groups around the shoulder strong to assist the rotator cuff in centering the humeral head on the glenoid.

Famed UFC coach Mike Winkeljohn, who helped shape UFC champion Jon Jones, Rashad Evans, and other famed fighters, notes the importance of stretching. "I think one of the most important parts of training is the warm-up. I think strikers don't stretch enough, especially their upper body. They also need to balance their upper-body training. Many of them do too many pushing exercises and not enough pulling exercises."

Many fighters are familiar with the military press and other exercises that work the large muscle groups of the shoulder region, but exercises for shoulder injury prevention need to focus on not only these big muscle groups, but also the smaller muscles, such as the rotator cuff. MMA veteran Renzo Gracie learned the value of resistance bands early on in his career and this lesson has stuck with him throughout the years. "At one point, I injured my shoulder. I couldn't raise my arm. When I went to raise my arm, it would lock. To rehab, I started using light weight and resistance bands, starting very slowly. I focused on stretching and motion and increasing blood flow to promote healing. I believe it's very important for fighters to use the resistance bands for their shoulders. It's just as important as the warm-up and cool-down. They are fabulous. Every day in the gym, the first thing I would do is warm up my shoulders, even before a treadmill run. My advice is to make it part of your regular routine and warm-up."

UFC Hall of Famer Mark Coleman echoes these sentiments, but reminds fighters that they have to actually put in the time. "Make sure to warm up your rotator cuff before training. There are great exercises out there, but you have to make sure you put in the time to warm up or to rehab." Cesar Gracie agrees that therapy bands are a great exercise. "You need to warm up to prevent shoulder injuries.

When you are going live, you need a sweat going. I know it's hard. These guys get in the gym and want to go right away. But you need to take the 20–30 minutes to get warm. Therapy bands are good, but unfortunately most people don't use them unless they have been injured."

UFC interim champion Carlos Condit follows a similar program for rotator cuff and shoulder warm-up. "We do rotator cuff work, lying on a bench with light dumbbells, rotating the arm with the elbows bent at 90 degrees. I also lift my arms in a 'Y' or 'W' using heavy bands, sitting with my back flush against the wall. I do my rotator cuff warm-up before almost every workout, especially on strength and conditions days."

# SHOULDER INJURY
# PREVENTION EXERCISES

It is important to emphasize both balanced strength and range of motion of the shoulders.

To work on range of motion, you can grab a broomstick or bar behind your back and move it out to either side.

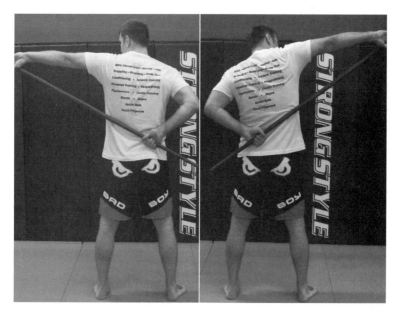

You can also raise the bar from in front over your head.

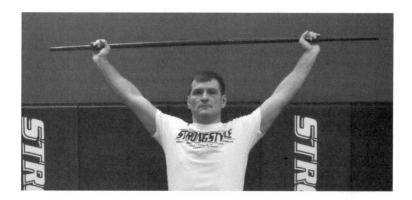

Simple movements help warm up and maintain range of motion. Resistance bands are a great way to warm up and strengthen your rotator cuff before a workout. Internal and external rotation at the side and up in the air work the different muscles of the rotator cuff.

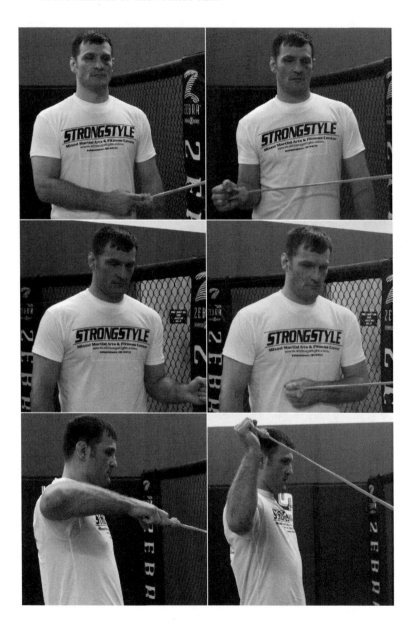

You can also use light weights while lying on your side, but be careful not to use too much weight so you isolate the rotator cuff in a safe manner.

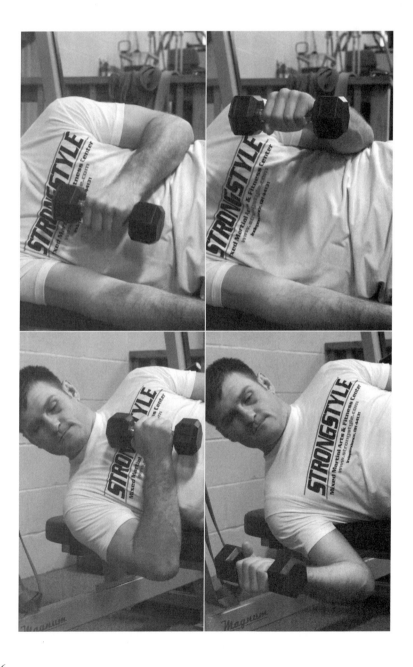

Lateral dumbbell raises

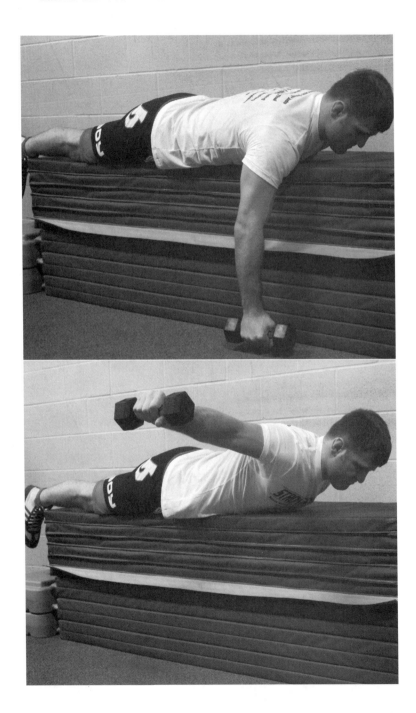

and squeezing your shoulder blades together helps coordinate the shoulder blade and the rest of your shoulder. This coordination helps reduce cuff and ligament injury.

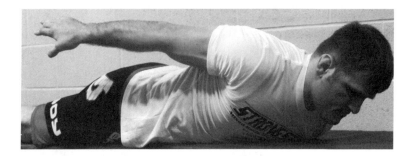

Many athletes develop tightness in the shoulders, especially in the back. Simple cross-body stretching

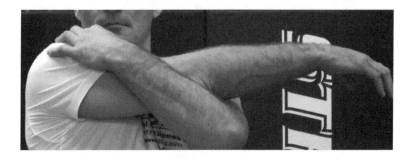

or the "sleeper" stretch can prevent you from developing too much tightness. Working the large muscles groups around the shoulder can help prevent the smaller muscle groups and ligaments from becoming stressed.

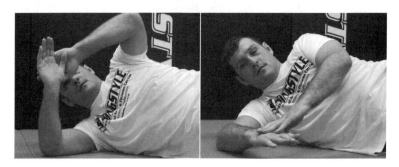

After a proper warm-up, start working in the larger muscle groups. The chest press is a good exercise for the pectoralis muscles.

You can also alternate arms on the incline press for a varied workout which emphasizes neuro-muscular control.

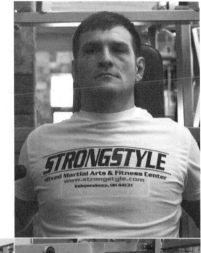

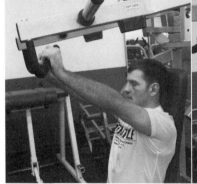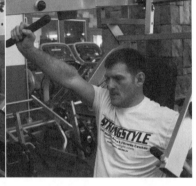

Reverse curls or "skull-crushers" work the triceps,

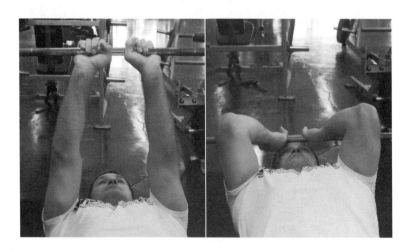

upright rows work the trapezius muscles,

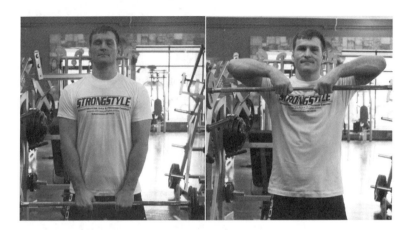

as do shoulder shrugs.

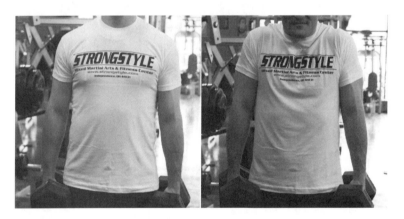

Seated rows help work the lattisimus dorsi muscles.

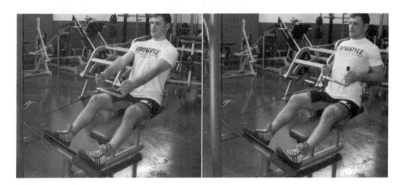

## CHAPTER 6

# HIP INJURIES AND
# "THE HAMMER'S" HIP

In 2008, Sean Sherk was training for his upcoming fight with BJ Penn when his right hip began to hurt. "The Muscle Shark" was known for his intense training routines, and it wasn't often something bothered him enough to have it checked out. He went to a doctor and underwent an MRI, which revealed a torn labrum. At the time, the UFC vet recalls, "Surgery wasn't an option." To help get through his training camp, Sean began to wear tight compression shorts, which provided extra support for his hip. "I like them so much, I even wear them while riding my snowmobile," says Sean.

## **ANATOMY**

The hip, like the shoulder, is a ball-and-socket joint. The socket is in the pelvis and is called the acetabulum. The ball is the top of the femur (thigh bone). Also, like the shoulder, it has a ring of cartilage called the labrum that circles the rim of the socket to help deepen and stabilize it. When a labrum tears, it can be very painful; however, more recent advances in orthopedic surgery have allowed labral tears

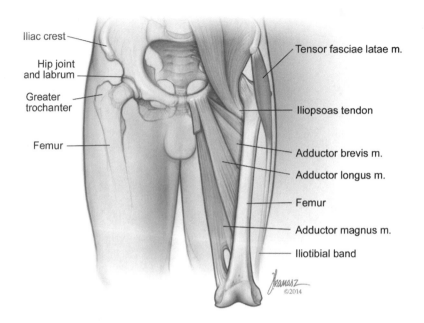

Iliac crest

Hip joint
and labrum

Greater
trochanter

Femur

Tensor fasciae latae m.

Iliopsoas tendon

Adductor brevis m.

Adductor longus m.

Femur

Adductor magnus m.

Iliotibial band

FRONT VIEW OF THE HIP SOCKET AND LABRUM WITH SOME OF THE
SURROUNDING MUSCLES THAT CAN GET INJURED. CREDIT: JOE KANASZ.

in young athletes to be repaired surgically using small arthroscopic
instruments.

Surrounding the hip joint are many large muscle groups including
the hip flexors (such as the iliopsoas); the quadriceps, which run over
the front of the thigh to the knee; the hamstrings in the back; the
adductors between the legs; and the abductors on the outside of the
leg. Any of these muscles can be injured due to a sudden trauma,
overuse, or generalized inflammation of the joint from other injuries.

## ADDUCTOR INJURIES

During his *UFC 100* fight with Thiago Alves, Georges St-Pierre went for
an arm-bar from his back during the fourth round. While attempting
the submission, he felt a tear in his groin and knew something was
wrong. With Alves raining shots down on him, GSP secured his guard
and wrapped Alves's arm to protect himself. The pain was so bad, GSP
began to pray that he make it through the round. Shortly after, GSP

managed to push Alves's hips back and stand back up. Despite suffering an adductor tear, he was able to stand back up and dominate the fight enough to win by unanimous decision.

The adductors are large muscles on the inner thigh that help bring the legs together. These muscles are especially important in a strong guard and a triangle choke. Like any muscle, both the meaty part of the muscle, called the "belly," and the tendon, which attaches the muscle to the bone, can be injured. Adductor strains, sometimes called "groin pulls," are particularly painful and can require months of rehab time. A doctor or certified athletic trainer can usually pinpoint the location of an adductor strain, but an MRI may be useful to rule out tears or complete tendon ruptures.

## SNAPPING HIPS

A snapping hip will affect many athletes, and it can be caused by several factors. Some aren't of any real concern and may just be from normal wear and tear, which can be the case with knee clicking as well. However, there are some causes that can be diagnosed and treated by a doctor. The first is the snapping of the iliotibial band, which runs along the outer side of your hip and leg. This thick band can snap over the greater trochanter, the sharp point on the side of the hip. Sometimes the sac around the greater trochanter can also get inflamed, leading to bursitis, which is an inflammation of the bursa sac — a lubricated cushion situated between a bone and the neighboring soft tissue.

Another cause of a snapping hip can be the iliopsoas muscles (hip flexors) sliding over the head of the femur. This is one of the most common causes of a snapping hip. Both of these causes of a snapping hip can usually be treated with rest and physical therapy. However, in the rare case where proper physical therapy doesn't work, surgery may be recommended.

The last cause of a snapping hip can be from a tear in the labrum. This can sometimes be treated with physical therapy, but if that fails, a surgeon may need to go into the hip arthroscopically and repair the labrum as well as shave off any bone prominences that may have led to the labral tear. UFC and Pride veteran Antônio Rodrigo Nogueira ended up requiring hip arthroscopies on both hips. His hips had bothered him for four years during his transition from Pride to the UFC, especially when he fought Randy Couture. The pain was so bad, he could barely sleep for four days before his fight with Couture. He would sit in ice baths to help with the pain. He would be late to training because his hips were so stiff in the morning. Eventually, "Minotauro" underwent surgery on both of his hips within a month of each other. However, despite having surgery on both hips, Minotauro managed to recover and fight seven months later in his hometown of Rio de Janeiro at *UFC 134*, defeating Brendan Schaub by KO in the first round.

## HAMSTRING RUPTURES

The hamstrings are the large muscle groups that run behind your leg and help you bend your knee. These can often be stretched with hyperextension by a knee bar or being kicked behind the leg. Sometimes, if the leg forcefully hyperextends, the hamstrings can rupture off of your ischial bone, which is the bone you sit on. If this happens, the fighter will experience an immense amount of pain and bruising of the entire leg. This can be treated with either surgery or rehab, and you should have a discussion with your surgeon regarding your recovery goals. Usually, a more active person will undergo surgery to maintain their active lifestyle and performance despite the long road of physical therapy and rehab after the surgery. A less active person can skip surgery and try to recover through rehab.

## INJURY PREVENTION

UFC Heavyweight Champion and Hall of Famer Mark Coleman suffered hip trauma that may have caused the need for early hip replacements. He also points out what orthopedic doctors know, but patients may not be aware of — that pain from the hip joint may actually be felt as groin pain or knee pain. It's important that you seek medical advice as soon as you feel any pain — there's always a chance it's a symptom of something more serious and harmful. As Coleman recalls, "In hindsight, it was an accumulation of getting my hips hurt on a daily basis. I didn't know I had an actual hip injury until I got images of my hip. The pain would be in my groin or my knee. I didn't want to go in and hear bad news. I wanted to try and get every fight out of me before someone pulled the plug. I was very lucky. I got hurt wrestling many times, but nothing that didn't heal up. Then I entered MMA. The wear and tear over the years and then getting older added up. The pain was there, but I dealt with it. I would just focus on making it to my next fight. Eventually, all my cartilage was gone and I needed a hip replacement. I was 44 years old my last fight. I always thought I would keep fighting or at least teach a long, long time. When you go into a fighting career, you need to keep in mind that something may end up hurting you long-term and something may end up nailing the coffin shut. As an athlete, I failed to get the proper x-rays. When you don't have the time or money to see the doctors, it's hard to get good care. Once I had the replacement, my knee didn't hurt anymore, my back didn't hurt anymore. My hip felt great. It would be ideal for any young fighter coming up to have good insurance so they can see doctors on a regular basis. And take advantage of it. Go see your doctor."

Ken Shamrock has had his fair share of hip injuries and recovery efforts, and he knows a fighter's "power comes from the center of their body and [an injury] takes away their ability to generate power and drive." It's easy for these injuries to be made worse without adequate rest and rehab at the first signs of pain.

In his experience as a world champion grappler and co-founder of American Top Team, Ricardo Liborio has noticed that the wrestlers like Mark Coleman who come to train are more susceptible to hip injuries than their jiu-jitsu based counterparts. "I believe wrestling causes a lot of hip injuries, more than jiu-jitsu. A lot of it probably comes from the sprawl. I think we have less hip injuries at ATT, because we are more jiu-jitsu based."

Since it's common for hips to get tight with wrestling and striking, a fighter has to work to prevent them from getting overdeveloped. As Frank Shamrock understands, "I have to consciously keep my hips and IT band relaxed and stretched. I use a foam roller every morning down my back and hips to help loosen up. I consciously release points of tension." Remember that tight muscles can make you predisposed to injuries, so keep relaxed and limber.

Like many other fighters, Gilbert Melendez echoes Shamrock's antidote: "I also work on my flexibility, especially after kicking. I like the butterfly stretch, doing splits at all angles, and while doing the splits, rotating my toes and body. I also like dynamic stretching, kicking my legs up and back, and also facing the wall and doing pendulum swings with my legs." One of Gilbert's coaches, Cesar Gracie has noticed that hip injuries tend to occur more with throws. "In my experience, hip injuries usually occur with judo throws. It's usually an injury to the hip flexors. When your hip flexors hurt, you need to really focus on stretching and deep massage such as acupressure. Some of our guys, like Nick Diaz, are good at hip stretching every day. Because he keeps his hips loose, his kicks are more fluid and it takes less effort to get his kicks off the ground."

Some hip injuries come from direct impact with your opponent and the ground, especially with judo-type throws. Understanding what surfaces you are falling onto and how to properly fall is something Carlos Newton instills in all of his students. "As a martial artist, you have to learn how to fall and pay attention to your body position whenever you are going to fall or get thrown. And know when to stop or yield. I knew I wanted to do martial arts for a long time — until I was an old man. I realized if I wanted to go down that long road, I needed to avoid training in new places I wasn't familiar with. If you are at a new gym or venue, you may have felt that the mats were cushy when you walked in, but when you get thrown on them, you feel they don't actually absorb the impact well. I suggest you walk around and get to know the place, get to know the mats, and get to know your surroundings. Develop a relationship with the mat and know if it literally has your back when the time comes. Don't let people peer pressure you into going harder or training in an uncomfortable position. Look them in the eye and say you will be back tomorrow. I pass these messages on to my students.

In my experience, jigsaw puzzle mats are not good for high impact. I like conventional judo mats. But also ask what's below the mats, what kind of surface is the mat on. Is it on a wood-frame floor with some deflection or something much harder? Careful selection of floors matters. Judo mats on a concrete floor may actually be worse than jigsaw mats on a wood floor."

# HIP STRENGTH AND
# FLEXIBILITY EXERCISES

Maintaining flexibility and range of motion in hips is important, especially for wrestlers.

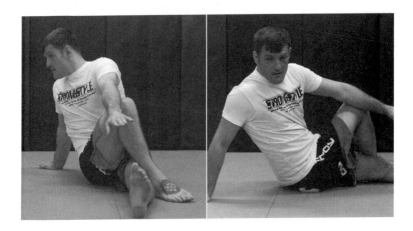

You can stretch the lateral structures, including the IT band with rotational movements.

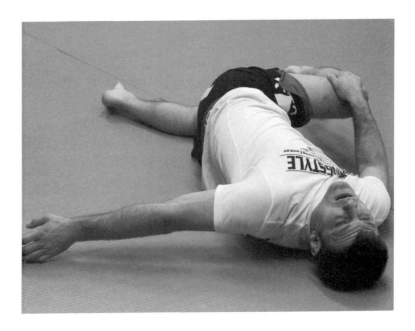

Stretch the front of the hip by placing your knee on a mat or block and slowly walking your front leg forward into a deep lunge.

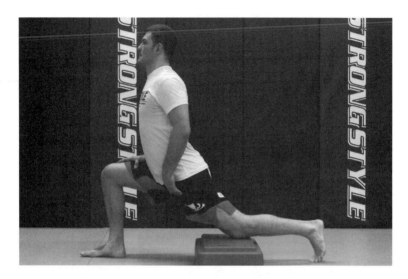

A foam roller on the side or front of the hip can help with recovery and soreness.

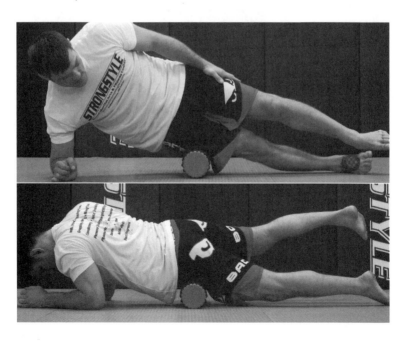

Plank and lateral posting exercises help your core but you can also add leg raises to increase the workload and bring your hip muscles into the equation.

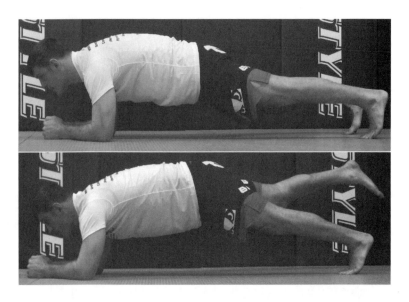

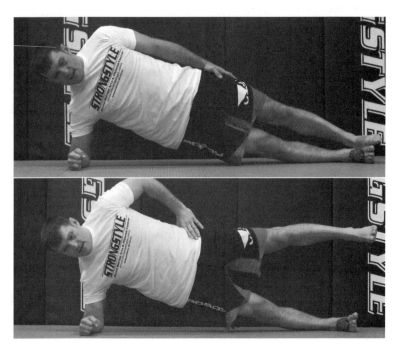

A partner can hold your legs while you slowly lower to the ground for eccentric exercises, which both stretch and strengthen the muscles.

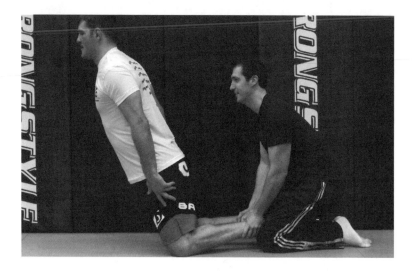

Eccentric exercises throughout the body are good workouts for tendonitis. Alternating arms and legs helps establish coordination.

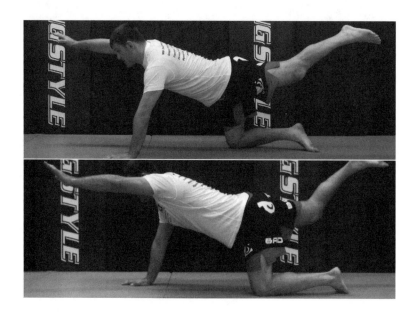

Pelvic lifts work the lower muscles,

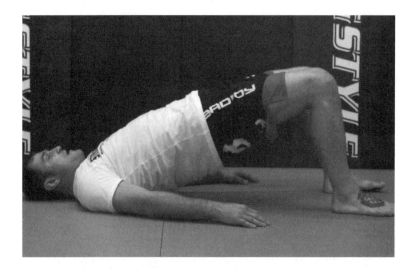

while adding a leg raise at the end really gives you a workout.

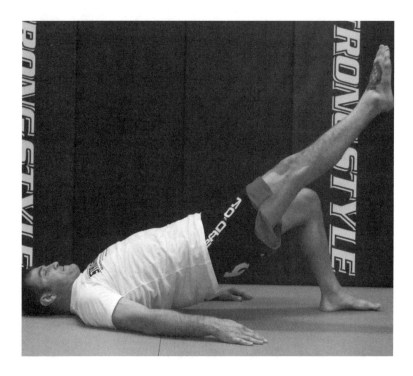

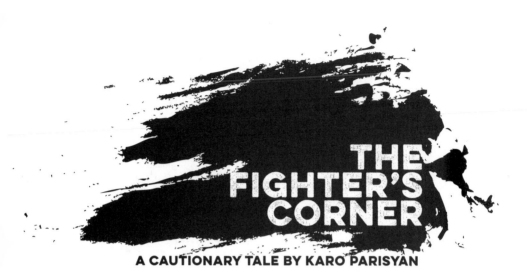

# THE FIGHTER'S CORNER

## A CAUTIONARY TALE BY KARO PARISYAN

My hamstring injury happened around 2005–2006. I had a six-fight win streak going and had gotten a title fight versus the champion Matt Hughes. I was training with Jason "Mayhem" Miller, Quinton "Rampage" Jackson, and Tito Ortiz. We were pretty warm and had a sweat going, but I didn't stretch out. I never really focused on that.

We all started grappling with each other. I gave Mayhem my back and he got his hooks in, so I stood up. He leaned over and tried to grab my ankle and foot. I resisted, and suddenly I felt and heard a "pop." Everyone thought I broke my femur. I fell down in shock. I almost threw up from the pain.

At the time I had a stick shift so I drove one and a half hours in L.A. traffic in agonizing pain. I went home, fell asleep, and woke up with everyone concerned. I started to get concerned that it was more than a pulled muscle. I went to a specialist, who thought I had a bad muscle pull and prescribed Vicodin.

I still hadn't dropped out of the fight. We went to Vegas and started training more for the fight. I tried to throw

Manny Gamburyan and fell flat on my face from the pain. Manny and I went back to the hotel and I got undressed to take a shower, and Manny, my cousin, said there was something wrong with my leg. The whole back of my leg was black and blue. Fifteen minutes later Dana White called me to ask about the injury, and I told him I had never pulled out of a fight. I didn't know what to do. Dana sent a driver to take me to the doctor, who examined me and told me I have a hamstring tear.

The doctor said I could treat my injury with either surgery or physical therapy. Dana thought surgery would be better and the UFC would cover it. I didn't like surgery and I didn't want to pull out of the fight. Eventually, the pain started to get so bad I couldn't tie my shoes. I ended up not fighting Matt Hughes.

I got a fight eight weeks later to Nick Thompson. Randy Couture was in my corner and I won in the first round. But the pain continued, and a huge ball of scar tissue started to form. I didn't do any rehab and didn't seek out any good advice. I didn't know what to do and eventually got very depressed. This led to my addiction to pain killers and putting my career in the toilet. Even today, I don't have the motion in my leg and often get shooting pain from the scar tissue.

I can't stress this enough, if you have a serious injury and you don't do anything about it, it will mess you up. I used to jump from my knees into an arm-bar, and I could tap a guy in no time. There is no way I can do that now. My right leg can hamstring curl 145 pounds, my injured leg can barely get 40 pounds. I still roll and submit people, but it's not the same. I had to change the way I do almost everything. You need to treat an injury before it's too late. Like my father says, you need to mold the metal while the iron is hot.

You should seek out good advice. For the injury I had, if you have the time and money, you can either do surgery or you can take the time to do the therapy right. Before this injury, I never took any pills in my life. I remember when I was a kid, my mom used to have to dissolve the pills for me since I was afraid of choking. At my worst I was swallowing 10 pills at once. Not taking care of an injury and not getting good information can be the beginning of the end. It's like a car; if you leave it alone, it will end up getting worse, costing more money, and other parts of the car will start to fall apart. Treat your body the right way. I found this out the hard way. One injury can end your entire career. It's part of the sport, but it comes with the package. There are a lot of ways to deal with injuries other than medication. If you have an injury, treat it the right way and don't focus on pain medication. Take it in moderation, only if you have to. It's very addictive stuff. It can rip your life apart. Time will heal your pain. The pills won't heal your injury. Healing comes with nutrition, doctors, and therapy.

If you are involved in any sport, especially mixed martial arts, you need to warm up. There is a reason coaches have been teaching students to warm up for 1,000 years. You need to warm up. You need to be sweating from your stretching in the gym, especially before grappling. Do it in a safe, active way. I never believed it until I got hurt. For my warm-up, I like 10 minutes of jumping rope, then gradually more stretching until all your muscles are warmed. No one is superhuman. We are not made from iron — you need to treat your body with respect.

## CHAPTER 7

# HAND INJURIES AND MAKING
# APPLESAUCE BARE-HANDED

To the untrained, boxing gloves are worn to protect an opponent's head from the battering of punching fists. In reality, it's the hands that need protecting. The hand contains some of the smallest and weakest bones in the body, which strike one of the hardest bones in the body, the cranium. When a punch occurs with enough impact, it's the small bones of the hand that usually fail (some areas of the facial bones are thinner, and thus they may fracture as well). According to veteran UFC trainer Mark DellaGrotte, hand injuries are some of the most common injuries he sees in his fighters. This chapter will focus on the more common broken bones and dislocations in the hand.

## ANATOMY

The vast majority of hand injuries that occur with striking sports are either fractures or dislocations. Based on the location of these injuries, treatment may be quite different. If you look at the back of your hand, you will see three sets of knuckles. The first row of knuckles, which is what most people strike with, is where the fingers attach

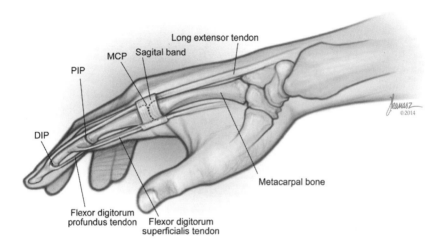

SIDE VIEW OF THE FINGER JOINTS AND MAJOR TENDONS.
CREDIT: JOE KANASZ.

to the palm. This is called the metacarpophalangeal (MCP) joint, because it is where the metacarpal bones (the bones that make up the non-finger part of the hand) attach to the phalangeal bones (the finger bones). The other two rows are called the proximal interphalangeal (PIP) joint and the distal interphalangeal (DIP) joint. The PIP joint is in the middle of the finger, while the DIP joint is closer to the fingernail.

## HAND FRACTURES

Martial arts experts have long known that one of the safest methods of punching is with a straight fist that strikes with the MCP joints of the index and middle fingers. These bones are larger than the other metacarpal bones and are more stable. Inadvertent striking with the small finger knuckle (MCP) either due to poor technique, fatigue, or looping punches can often result in a fracture. This type of injury has been nicknamed "the boxer's fracture" due to its frequent occurrence among boxers.

## TREATMENT

A boxer's fracture or other metacarpal fractures can be very angulated and should be x-rayed and realigned by a professional. Once it is realigned, it must be immobilized in a splint or cast to prevent the angular deformity from occurring before the bone heals. Once the bone heals, there may be a residual bump, but the function of the hand should not be compromised, unless there is a large degree of deformity. If, however, the alignment of the bone cannot be maintained in a splint or cast, a doctor may offer surgery to hold the bone in place with hardware. Hardware may include small screws, a plate and screws, or removable pins placed percutaneously (poked through the skin and drilled into the bone). Fractures between the MCP joint and the PIP joint are often treated in the same manner. This is in contrast to fractures in between the PIP joint to the tip of the finger, as these often do not need surgery. They may need to be realigned with some traction by a professional, but they generally can be buddy taped to the neighboring finger for support.

If a healthcare professional recommends a splint or cast, it should be respected. Once the injury heals, then it will be acceptable to begin a gentle range of motion to overcome the stiffness that may have developed. It's always better to need therapy for stiffness than to not have a bone or ligament heal properly, which draws the pain out even longer.

If you must continue to train striking technique, there are ways to minimize the pain while training. Josh Barnett trains using the uninjured hand at full power but modifies the other hand accordingly: "One time, I had a training partner and his hand was bothering him, so I worked with him around it. If you throw your hurting power hand, I will make sure to act like it's not hurt. You can throw it with less power and I will treat it like it's being thrown with full power. Another thing is, if your knuckles are sore, try some gel padding as a shock absorber. I have found them to work pretty well."

UFC champion Demetrious Johnson felt the effects of a metacarpal fracture very early in his career. "My very first injury as an amateur was a broken hand," recalls Demetrious. "The doctors had to pin my index finger metacarpal. Since I was working full-time at a warehouse job, I rehabbed myself. After I got the pin out, I started back slowly. But even when I hit, I could feel the bone rattle. With hand injuries, it's all about where and how you hit. With my injury, I hit a guy in the head, and the small bone lost to the big bone. To help prevent hand injuries, I wear 16 oz gloves for sparring, so I can protect myself and my training partners. I wear 7 oz gloves for MMA. You should try and pad up as much as you can."

### FINDING THE CONFIDENCE TO HIT HARD AGAIN

Tim Silvia has experienced firsthand the long physical and mental recovery hand fractures can sometimes take. He knows one of the hardest things for a fighter to overcome after a hand injury, even after it's healed, is confidence — the confidence to start throwing hard punches again. "I have had plates put on the ring finger metacarpals of both hands. As part of my rehab, I squeezed tennis balls to work on my grip strength. It took about six months of training before I felt confident in throwing hard again. Usually I use 18 oz gloves, but after getting hurt, I was using 24 oz until I had the confidence to go back down to 18 oz."

Cesar Gracie, coach to many top-level UFC fighters, recommends getting hand fractures realigned by a doctor for two reasons: psychological and physical. "With a deformed broken bone, there is a psychological aspect that bothers the fighter — you tend to not throw as hard with that deformed hand. You don't want that limitation during a fight. And in my experience, they tend to break easier again when they heal at an angle. It's a traumatic experience when you break something. The pain is sent searing through your whole body. To help prevent injury, you want a professional wrapping your hands. In competition, we prefer both cloth and tape for wrapping. In training we do Mexican-style elastic wraps."

According to Frank Shamrock, if you're an MMA athlete and "you got no hands, you got nothing." This can make hand injuries a real wake-up call to those who don't take the care to protect their hands. In order to make sure you prevent hand injuries, he recommends two things: wrap your hands and punch with the first two knuckles. Not only does wrapping protect your bones and tendons, it also keeps your hands and wrists strong.

Frank Shamrock continues, "Maintaining a weightlifting regimen keeps my hands and wrists strong. I focus on the muscles that support my hands and wrists. I like exercises that use just hands, like climbing trees. Most people don't understand why they wrap their hands. It's to keep everything aligned and distribute the force. I spent the first 10 years of my career punching without wraps until I realized your hands are a limited resource."

Carlos Newton also understands the importance of building up technique and the appropriate muscles to support your hands in striking. "The biggest mistake guys make when they start training is they buy wraps and boxing gloves and start hitting hard right away. Don't do that. Start without gloves and wraps and learn how to make a proper fist and have proper technique and alignment. You need to develop these and train lightly to get a feel for balance. My boxing coach has taught me a lot. They say when the pupil is ready, the master will appear. Once you reach a certain level, it's no longer a question of technique, it then becomes a matter of force. Then you need to glove up and strike hard in practice. If you have bad technique and form and you have only trained with big gloves, then when you go to use the smaller 6 oz MMA gloves, you will get hurt."

### WORKING ON GRIP STRENGTH

Frank's adopted brother and UFC Hall of Famer Ken Shamrock also experienced a hand injury and touts the importance of hand exercises: "Before my second fight with Tito Ortiz, I was training and blocked a kick with my hand and the kick bent my fingers back. Then I threw a

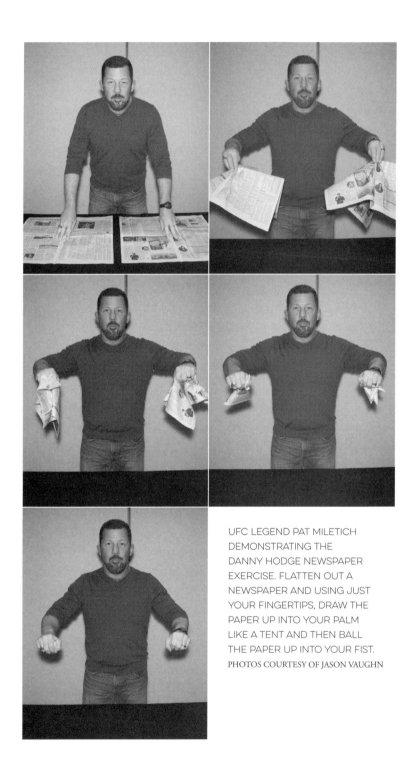

UFC LEGEND PAT MILETICH DEMONSTRATING THE DANNY HODGE NEWSPAPER EXERCISE. FLATTEN OUT A NEWSPAPER AND USING JUST YOUR FINGERTIPS, DRAW THE PAPER UP INTO YOUR PALM LIKE A TENT AND THEN BALL THE PAPER UP INTO YOUR FIST.
PHOTOS COURTESY OF JASON VAUGHN

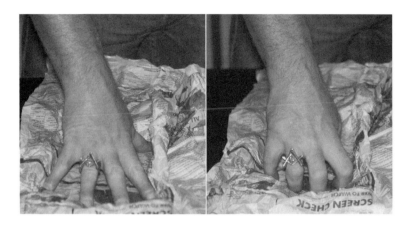

CLOSE-UP OF HOW THE FINGERS DRAW UP THE NEWSPAPER.

punch, and I broke my first and second metacarpals. I was treated with a cast. To rehab, I did a lot of grip work like squeezing play-dough and grabbing the edge of a newspaper to bring the newspaper into a ball."

The newspaper ball exercise is actually a well-known exercise among professional grapplers and wrestlers. Retired MMA fighter Pat Miletich recalls hearing stories of a legendarily strong Olympic wrestler named Danny Hodge, who could make applesauce with his bare hands. "I first met Danny Hodge in Oklahoma. I asked him how he got such legendary grip strength and he showed me the newspaper exercise. He said to lay two pages flat on top of each other and then grab them between fingers in the middle of the square and make a little tent. Then gradually ball up a page in each hand. Then unfold them, straighten them, and repeat. I would do it three times a day."

American Top Team co-founder and jiu-jitsu champion Ricardo Liborio also sees a role for grip strength, especially when practicing grappling with a gi (a traditional martial arts uniform). "There is no doubt that working on your grip helps prevent injuries, especially in jiu-jitsu. What happens in jiu-jitsu is you get the fingers caught in the gi and twisted. Or when guys hold your fingers to try and break a submission attempt. I remember, I was fighting a Japanese opponent in the ADCC [Abu Dhabi Combat Club] tournament and he grabbed my finger and caught it and broke it right away. To work on your grip strength, I have seen gi fabric attached to a string attached to a weight machine. Or you can wrap your gi over a pull-up bar and practice pulling yourself up by grabbing the gi."

UFC champion Carlos Condit has used several exercises to keep his hands strong. "I definitely like ice for healing, and for grip strength, we use weighted sleds and ropes. Sometimes we fill a bucket with rice, and I put my hand in rice and use it for resistance. You can work on grabbing, pinching, and turning your hand in the rice. I also do pull-ups holding a towel over a pull-up bar to work on different grips. I have also done a little bit of rock climbing for fun and grip strength."

Don "The Predator" Frye, an MMA veteran, shares a story to remind fighters that protecting your hands needs to happen both inside and outside the cage. Simply put, getting into fights outside the cage can result in a hand fracture, and as Frank mentioned, your hands are a limited resource. "I remember I first broke my hand against Tank Abbott in the finals when I won the *Ultimate Ultimate* tournament. Back then, they just wrapped the back of the hand. They didn't wrap the knuckles like they should have. The tape ended before the knuckles. We know better now. But unfortunately, I broke it again one year later. I was walking out a bar with fellow UFC fighter Brian Johnston. At *UFC 10* we were opponents, but we became friends. We have been good friends since then. At some point, we were leaving a bar and some guy was messing with a girl. I fractured my hand due to an altercation. The first time it broke, it was fixed with pins, but the second time it had to be fixed with a plate. Now I wrap my hands all the time and spar with 18–20 oz gloves to protect my hands as much as possible."

## FINGER DISLOCATIONS AND FRACTURES

Besides fractures, finger dislocations can occur. With the use of fingerless MMA gloves, the incidence of dislocations is higher than in boxing. Dislocations can be either simple or complex. Simple dislocations often can be reduced and immediate range of motion

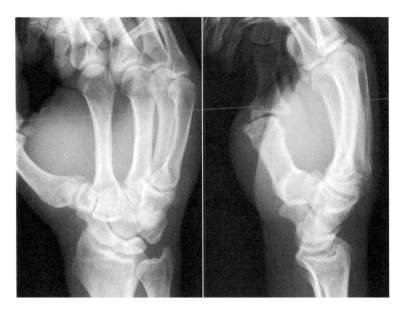

X-RAYS OF KEN SHAMROCK'S HAND SHOWING AN AVULSION OF A PIECE OF BONE AT THE BASE OF THE THUMB MCP JOINT (LEFT IMAGE) AND A PARTIAL DISLOCATION OF THE THUMB IP (INTERPHALANGEAL) JOINT (RIGHT IMAGE). PHOTO COURTESY OF KEN SHAMROCK.

performed. Complex dislocations, however, may involve rupture of ligaments or fractures, neither of which can be confirmed without proper x-rays and examination. While the instinct of a fighter may be to just pull on a dislocation and not seek medical treatment, it is very easy for a finger injury to lead to pain and stiffness if not treated properly. Ken Shamrock has suffered several ligament injuries on his thumb, which have led to chronic instability of his thumb joints. Ken recalls one of his injuries. "I was in the middle of training and blocked a kick with my hand. The kick caught my thumb and pushed it backwards towards my wrist. I taped it and finished training. However, it ended up swelling a lot and becoming stiff. In hindsight, I wish I had seen a doctor!" If you look at Ken's first hand x-ray, you can see a fleck of bone at the base of his thumb metacarpal that was pulled away by his ligament — this is often referred to as a "skier's thumb" or "gamekeeper's thumb" depending on whether it's acute (skier's) or chronic. In the second x-ray looking at his hand

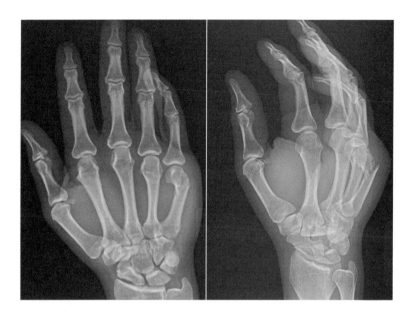

FRONT AND OBLIQUE VIEW OF A FIFTH (SMALL FINGER) METACARPAL
NECK FRACTURE, ALSO KNOWN AS A "BOXER'S FRACTURE."
PHOTO COURTESY OF THE AUTHOR

from the side, you can see the joint above the other injury is not completely lined up, because of his non-reduced partial dislocation.

Gilbert Melendez has developed a small technique change to try to avoid getting your fingers caught and bent into awkward positions. "A lot of the time in MMA, your hands are loose while grappling and your fingers can get caught. You can't keep your hands tight like in boxing, so it's easy to get a knuckle caught. My advice is to always tape your hands and always be aware of your position. Keep your hands in a fist or tense in a flexed position. Stay loose for flow but keep them ready to tense up at any time. This goes for all of your body. When you throw a punch, you start loose then tense up. Your kicks start light and then snap at the end. The same idea holds for your hands. Keep them loose for flow, but be ready to tighten them up quickly."

## TENDON INJURIES

Other hand injuries a fighter may encounter are ligament and tendon ruptures. Ligaments are strong ropes of tissue that connect

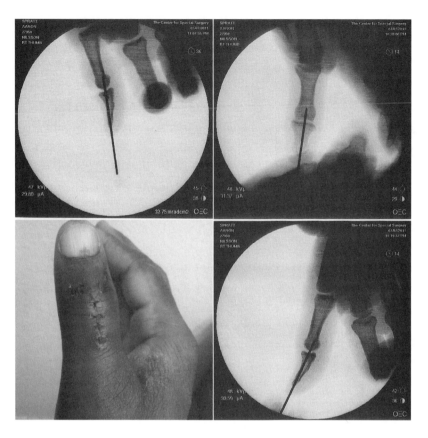

INTRA-OPERATIVE AND POST-OPERATIVE VIEWS OF PETE SPRATT'S FINGER AFTER PINNING THE IP JOINT. PHOTO COURTESY OF PETE SPRATT.

two bones together. Tendons are the ends of muscles that attach to bones to move them. The tendons on the top of the hand that allow the fingers to extend are called extensor tendons and the tendons on the bottom of the hand that flex the fingers are called flexor tendons. Sometimes due to a sudden pull or twist, tendons or ligaments can rupture. While some of these ruptures can be treated with strict immobilization using a splint, many others will need surgery. If you rupture a tendon, you should seek medical treatment within a week.

If the extensor tendon ruptures from its insertion at the tip of the finger, it is called a "mallet finger," since the tip of the finger bends, and it looks like a mallet. If the flexor tendon is ruptured off the tip of the finger, it's called a "jersey finger," since it is often caused when a player is grabbing another player's jersey and the jersey is suddenly pulled away. In both cases, a doctor will need to examine the fighter and get x-rays to determine whether a splint or surgery is the proper treatment. A third common hand injury in MMA is called a "boxer's knuckle." In this injury, the hood that holds the extensor tendon over the MCP knuckle ruptures and allows the tendon to move to the side of the knuckle, especially when a fist is made. This can lead to the extensor tendon not working as it should and preventing the fighter from fully extending the finger. This is often treated with a splint, but sometimes surgery is necessary to repair the extensor tendon hood.

MMA veteran Pete Spratt explains his injury, "The biggest injury I have sustained in 13 years of fighting has to be the ruptured thumb tendon. I remember feeling a pain in my thumb in the first round and when I came back to my corner in between rounds, I looked down at my thumb and it was pretty swollen!" Pete went on to have surgery to reattach one of the thumb extensor tendons and insert a pin to keep the thumb in place while the tendon healed.

### GIVING YOUR HANDS TIME TO HEAL

Renzo Gracie learned the hard way that not letting a hand injury heal only prolongs your downtime. "I hurt my hand fighting Oleg Taktarov in 1996. Back then it was bareknuckle. I didn't realize his head was so hard! It took six months for me to recover because I never rested it. I didn't stop training and was constantly looking to fight. Looking back, I would have stopped and let it heal. You can work around it. Run, do elliptical, do the bicycle. In the end I probably delayed my fighting by not properly resting it to heal it."

UFC Middleweight Champion Chris Weidman also felt the pain of a significant hand injury and wasn't able to let it heal until after his fight. Hands often get hurt, and fighters often do not pull out of fights for various reasons. If that's the case, make sure to give your hand the time it needs to heal after the fight. At *UFC 175*, Weidman successfully defended his UFC Middleweight Championship in five rounds against the always dangerous Lyoto Machida. But three weeks before the fight, Weidman suffered a thumb injury and was worried he would need to pull out of the match. His trainer Ray Longo remembers the story, "Weidman hurt his hand three weeks before the Machida fight. He got x-rays and an MRI. They showed a sprained ligament. The doctor told him it was injured, but wouldn't get worse. However, he couldn't use it. He couldn't throw a left hand. So we had to change up his game plan and Chris did more kicking. It was a high stakes fight, so I have to know my fighter. He wasn't going to pull out so we needed to find a new strategy. After the fight, it never got better. Even grazing the thumb would kill him. We ended up seeing a second doctor and getting more images. This time the doctor saw a hairline fracture, and he ended up needing a cast. After the fight, we were able to work around it and not cause any more stress on the thumb until it finally healed."

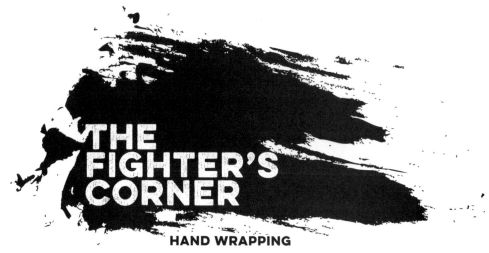

## THE FIGHTER'S CORNER

### HAND WRAPPING
WITH MARK DELLAGROTTE

According to Mark DellaGrotte the importance of proper hand wrapping cannot be overstated. "How we wrap fighters' hands can make or break careers. There are very few coaches who wrap hands. I do it because Stitch taught me. If it weren't for guys like him who know what they are doing, more careers would be ended. He actually calls me Grasshopper because of my interest in learning from him. Not only is it important to wrap the hands for fight night, but it's also important during training camp. Guys don't pay attention to this during training camp, and they suffer smaller injuries that predispose them to injury on fight night."

Legendary MMA and Brazilian Jiu-Jitsu expert Mario Sperry has some hand injury advice too, "Most of the time, hand injuries happen because a fighter is used to training by shadowboxing and is too relaxed with his open hands. This becomes especially true when they are tired. During the fight, you fight how you train, and the combination of small gloves, the extra force of a fight, and punching with open hands can be devastating."

And if you do hurt your hands, Mario has some more thoughts: "Always use ice right away and see a doctor. Whenever someone is recovering from a hand injury, I give them the advice that a famous Brazilian volleyball player gave to me: contrast. Hot and cold. Get two buckets. One with warm water and the other one with ice water. Stick your hand inside one then the other and alternate for a few minutes."

Former UFC champion Sean Sherk also recognizes the importance of hand wrapping and ice. "For the first six or seven years of my career, I never wrapped my hands. I was throwing a thousand punches a day on heavy bags, Muay Thai mitts, and ground and pound bags. My hands started hurting all the time. I was trying to be a tough guy. I don't know what I was thinking. I definitely should have been wrapping my hands."

Stitch, however, reminds everyone that while wraps are important, they don't make you invincible. "One thing I always tell people, because I have a very good wrap, is that a good wrap doesn't guarantee you won't break your hand. It minimizes the possibility of you breaking your hand, but a lot of these guys, especially in MMA, where they're throwing a lot of hooks and land on top of the head — there's no support factor when the knuckles make contact with the head. It's pretty easy to break your hand that way."

Coach Mike Winkeljohn echoes this statement. "Hand wraps are very important. Especially wrapping the thumbs to make the hand one unit makes a gigantic difference. But be careful with overhand punches. Overhands with the first knuckle are good if you can knock a guy out, but if you are too long with your punch and hit his head, you can really get hurt." Former professional fighter Andy Foster has seen fighters neglect hand wrapping and the resulting injuries. "I broke my right hand once. The trick to avoiding this is to make sure the wrapping used for sparring is consistent. In haste, sometimes we shortcut the wrapping process to get into the ring. This leads to hand injuries. Haste makes waste . . . and injuries."

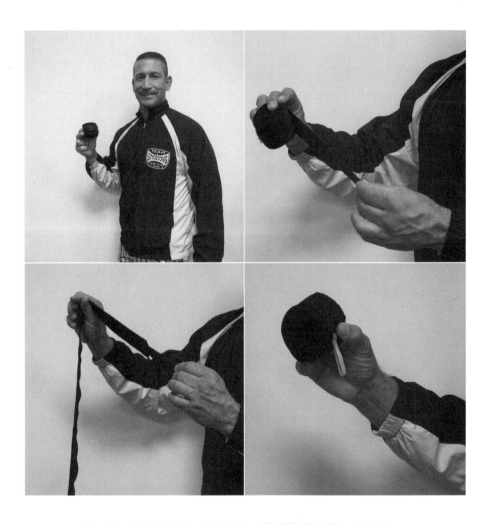

FOR NON-COMPETITION, MARK DELLAGROTTE PREFERS MEXICAN-STYLE HAND WRAPS, WHICH USE A MORE FLEXIBLE MATERIAL TO ALLOW FOR BETTER CIRCULATION. LONGER LENGTHS ARE USUALLY BETTER THAN SHORTER LENGTHS SO YOU DON'T RUN OUT OF MATERIAL. ONCE YOU TAKE IT OUT OF THE PACKAGE, UNROLL IT AND THEN ROLL IT BACK UP IN THE REVERSE DIRECTION STARTING WITH THE END THAT WAS ORIGINALLY ON THE OUTSIDE.

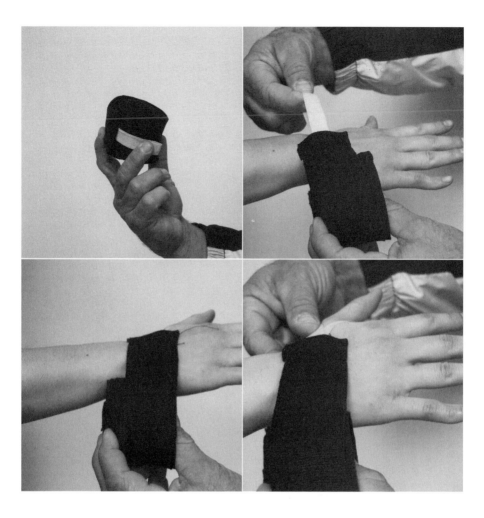

START BY PLACING THE THUMB IN THE THUMB LOOP, AND THEN BEGIN WRAPPING OVER THE BACK OF THE HAND, AWAY FROM THE THUMB. WRAP AROUND THE WRIST THREE TO FIVE TIMES DEPENDING ON THE SIZE OF THE HAND.

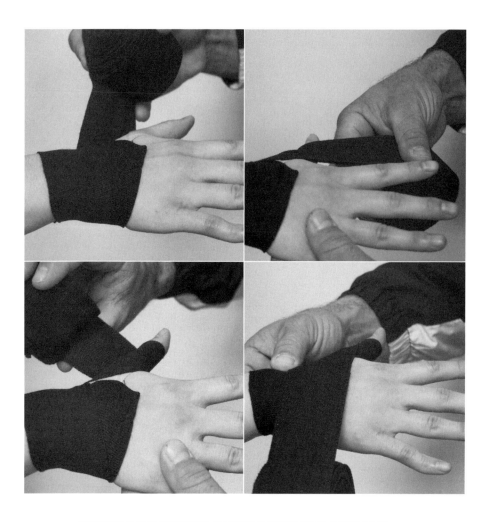

START ON THE THUMB SIDE. BRING THE WRAP OVER THE THUMB
TO THE SPACE BETWEEN THE INDEX FINGER AND THE THUMB,
WRAPPING AROUND THE THUMB, THEN ACROSS THE LOWER BACK
OF THE HAND (WHERE THE HAND MEETS THE WRIST) TO THE SMALL
FINGER SIDE. WRAP UNDER THE WRIST TO THE THUMB SIDE.
DO THIS TWO TO FIVE TIMES.

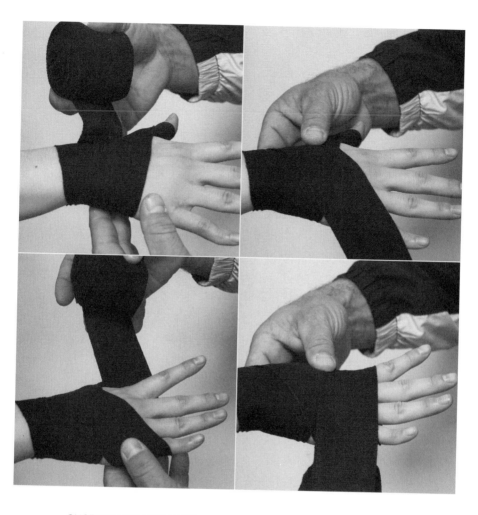

ONCE YOU ARE BACK AROUND TO THE THUMB SIDE, CROSS
DIAGONALLY OVER THE BACK OF THE HAND TO REACH THE OUTSIDE
OF THE LITTLE FINGER. THIS IS THE FIRST STEP OF WRAPPING THE
FINGERS TOGETHER AS A WHOLE.

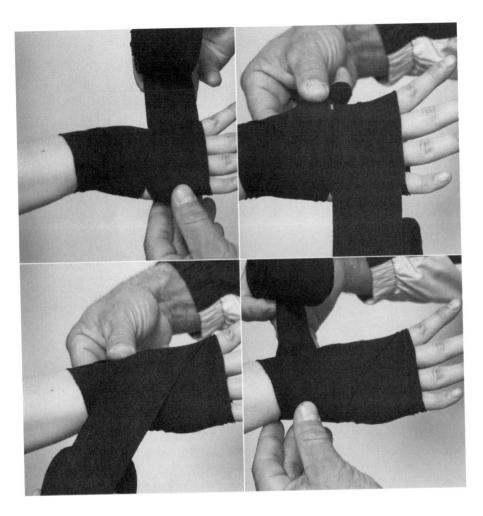

WRAP AROUND THE BASE OF THE FINGERS WITH THE FINGERS SPREAD WIDE THREE TO FIVE TIMES. THEN RETURN TO THE WRIST AND WRAP AROUND TO THE THUMB SIDE TO PREPARE FOR WRAPPING EACH FINGER INDIVIDUALLY.

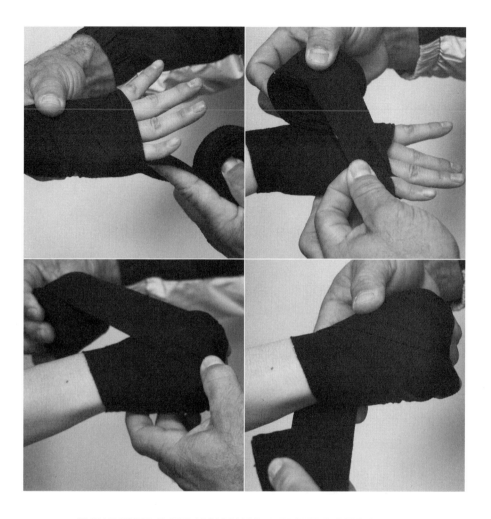

FROM THE THUMB SIDE CROSS DIAGONALLY OVER THE TOP OF
THE HAND AND WRAP THE SMALL FINGER BY PASSING ALONG THE
OUTSIDE, WRAPPING AROUND IT, MOVING IN BETWEEN THE SMALL
FINGER AND RING FINGER, AND THEN RETURNING TO THE THUMB
SIDE. OPEN THE HAND WHEN YOU PASS BETWEEN THE FINGERS,
THEN CLOSE THE HAND INTO A FIST WHEN YOU COME ACROSS THE
KNUCKLES, HEADING BACK TOWARDS THE WRIST. PASS THE WRAP
UNDER THE WRIST TO REACH THE SMALL FINGER SIDE.

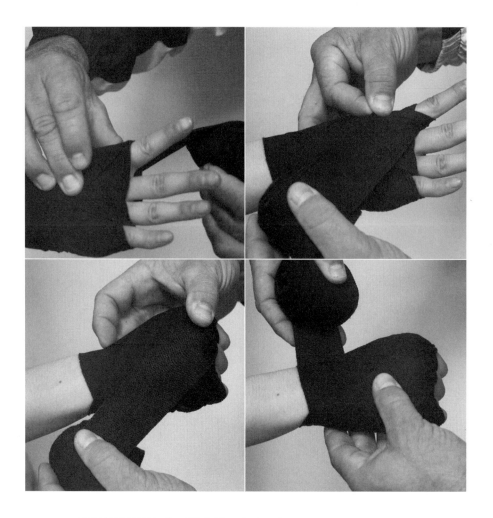

FROM THE SMALL FINGER SIDE, WRAP THE INDEX FINGER BY PASSING
OVER THE TOP OF THE WRIST TO THE THUMB SIDE OF THE FINGER,
WRAPPING UNDERNEATH THE INDEX FINGER THROUGH THE SPACE
BETWEEN THE INDEX FINGER AND THE THUMB, AND RETURNING
TO THE WRIST THROUGH THE INDEX AND MIDDLE FINGERS. WITH
EACH FINGER WRAP, YOU RETURN TO THE SAME SIDE YOU STARTED
WRAPPING THE FINGER FROM, THEN PASS UNDER THE WRIST TO
PREPARE FOR THE NEXT FINGER TO BE WRAPPED.

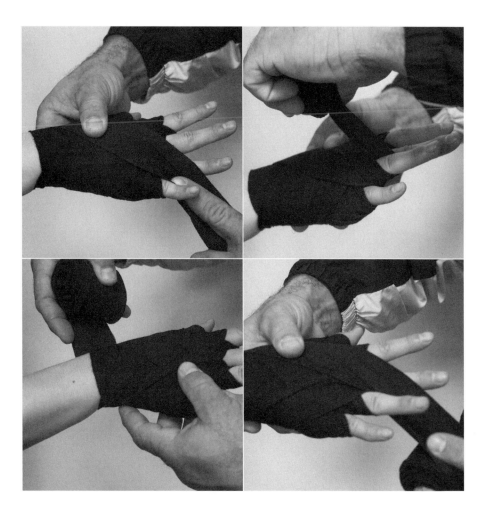

WRAP THE RING FINGER BY PASSING BETWEEN THE RING AND
SMALL FINGERS, WRAPPING AROUND THE RING FINGER TO COME
OUT BETWEEN RING AND MIDDLE, THEN RETURN TO THE THUMB
AND WRAP AROUND THE WRIST. THEN WRAP THE MIDDLE FINGER BY
PASSING BETWEEN INDEX AND MIDDLE FINGERS, WRAPPING AROUND
THE MIDDLE FINGER TO COME BACK OUT BETWEEN MIDDLE AND
RING. IT IS IMPORTANT TO MAKE SURE THERE IS NO BUNCHING OF
THE MATERIAL.

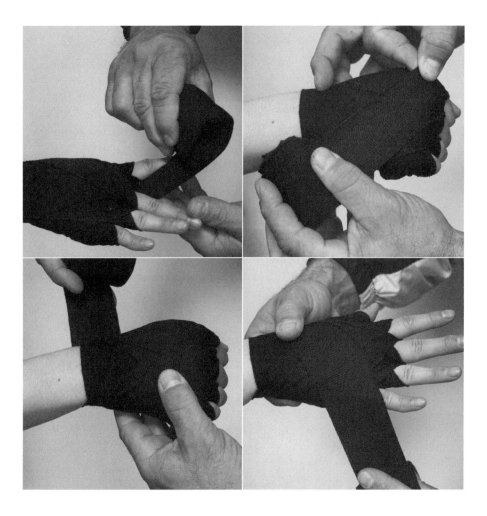

AFTER THE MIDDLE FINGER HAS BEEN WRAPPED, WRAP AROUND
THE WRIST ONE MORE TIME TO BRING THE WRAP BACK TO THE
KNUCKLES.

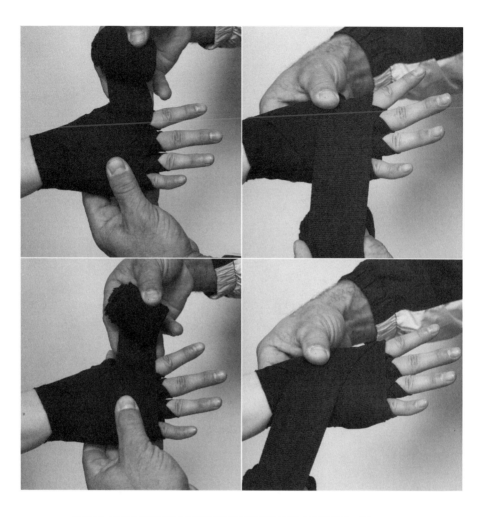

WRAP AROUND THE KNUCKLES ANOTHER TWO TO FIVE TIMES.

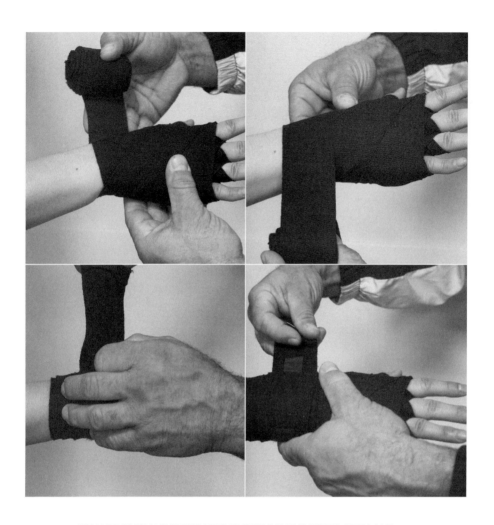

FINALLY, FINISH UP BY WRAPPING AROUND THE WRIST. OPEN AND CLOSE THE HAND TO MAKE SURE MATERIAL DOES NOT BUNCH UP OR CUT OFF CIRCULATION. EXAMINE ALL SIDES OF THE HAND.

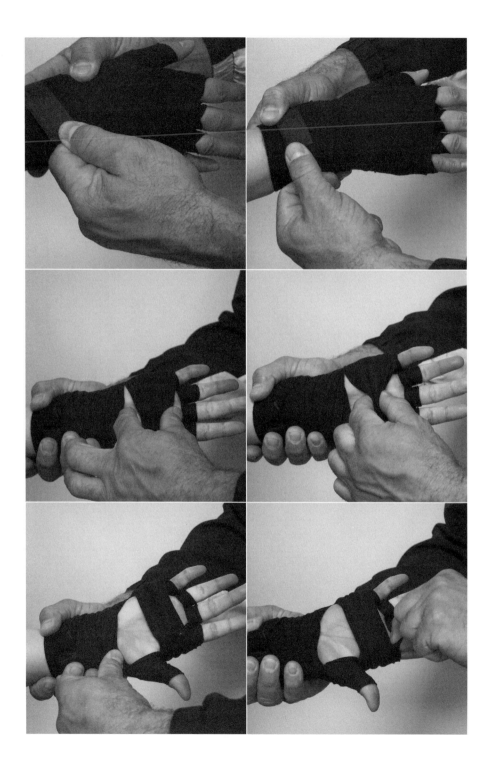

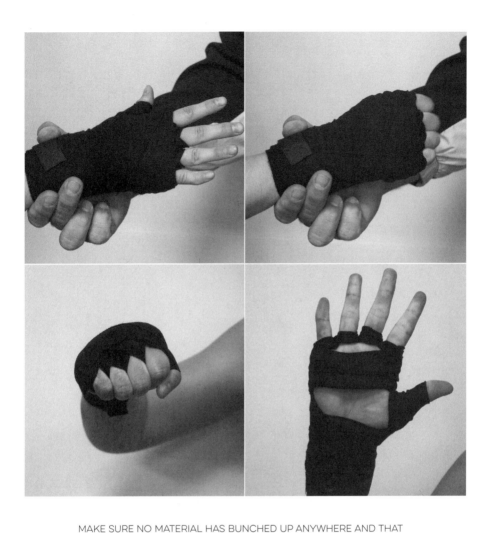

MAKE SURE NO MATERIAL HAS BUNCHED UP ANYWHERE AND THAT YOUR HAND HAS A FLEXIBLE RANGE OF MOTION AND PROPER BLOOD CIRCULATION. PHOTOS COURTESY OF RICHARD FOX

CHAPTER **8**
# SKIN INFECTIONS AND HOW
# MARK DELLAGROTTE SAVED *TUF*

Besides traumatic injuries, one particularly important issue that
sidelines mixed martial artists and other athletes is skin infections.
Ignoring skin infections and not seeing a trained medical professional places not only a fighter at risk, but also his entire team and
training partners. Sometimes, skin infections can become so severe
they can lead to hospitalization and even surgery. Recognizing some
of the more common athletic skin infections can go a long way in
both treatment and prevention.

## HERPES
The name herpes alone seems taboo for some athletes to discuss.
There is often a stigma tied to herpes that links it to sexually transmitted diseases. While some of the herpes viruses are contracted via
sexual contact, other types of herpes can be transmitted via skin-to-
skin contact. They are not the same exact viruses, but share similar
characteristics and are therefore grouped into the same family. In
fact, the chicken pox falls into this same herpes virus family. The
herpes virus often presents as a painful "cold sore" near the mouth

and lasts four or five days. Eventually, the fluid-filled blisters crust over and disappear, but anytime the body is stressed and the immune system defenses are lowered, the sores may return.

During the contagious stage before the blisters are crusted over, any skin-to-skin contact between training partners or opponents can lead to infection. The site of infection isn't limited to around the mouth. Cheeks or even fingers can become infected with herpes sores. The common association with wrestling and grapplers has even led to the term herpes gladiatorum, a reference to the Roman gladiators. While the condition is permanent, some medications help prevent or treat outbreaks. This is something to speak to your doctor about.

## IMPETIGO

Staph infections are a common term thrown around locker rooms. Impetigo is a bacterial infection caused by two types of bacteria: staphylococcus (staph for short) and streptococcus (strep for short). When there is a break in the skin, even microscopic, sometimes the bacteria can get by the barrier and cause a skin infection. Impetigo is highly contagious and appears as a yellowish blister that leads to a honey-colored scab. Proper hygiene can help prevent its spread, and if a fighter is infected, proper antibiotics prescribed by a doctor can easily treat the infection. Studies have also shown that the best way to prevent spread is to keep infected skin lesions covered.

Demetrious Johnson had a bout with impetigo, and as a result, his training camp suffered. "My training partner had impetigo. He then gave it to me. Shortly after, I shaved my beard and it made it worse. It finally cleared up in about 10 days with antibiotics. It was the worst week of my training camp — really messed with my cardio."

MRSA is one particular type of staph infection. MRSA stands for Methicillin-resistant Staphylococcus aureus, which means it's a staph infection that is resistant to common medications similar to penicillin. This particular strain is becoming more common in the community, and it can spread quickly; therefore, prompt attention by a trained medical professional is important to prevent things from going from bad to worse. Sometimes it looks just like a small pimple, but that just may be the tip of the iceberg. The contents of entire NFL locker rooms have needed to be torn apart and rebuilt after falling under colonization from staph infections.

Staph infections are so pervasive that they almost brought an entire *Ultimate Fighter* season to a grinding halt. Mark DellaGrotte recalls his experience working with the fighters on *The Ultimate Fighter*: "About eight to 10 years ago, we started to see a lot of guys get staph infections in the gyms. It was a real problem. I was coaching season four of *TUF*. It was called 'The Comeback' show. They had me as a coach along with Georges St-Pierre, Randy Couture, and Marc Laimon. Edwin Dewees and another guy had some funny looking pimples on their body. I saw them and thought they looked suspicious for staph. I brought it to the attention of the staff and we went to the hospital, and it was in fact staph. I told Dana White to watch out for all of the cast to get it. This was a serious issue and could end the show if all of the cast members got it. And sure enough, one by one, everyone got it.

"Everyone at the UFC and the TV producers began to get worried. So I looked into how they cleaned the equipment. I asked if they sanitized the mats and they said 'Yes, we clean the mats everyday.' I then asked if they cleaned the walls too and they asked, 'Why?' Well, the walls were padded with mats, so they needed to be cleaned like the floor mats. These fighters are training shirtless and they are constantly rubbing their backs up and down against the wall. I asked them if they ever cleaned the wall mats in the last four seasons? Not once. How about the stability balls? No. So none of the equipment except the floor mats were cleaned for four seasons. I advised them to clean everything. Even the canvas needs to be changed after each event, regardless of whether the sponsors had changed. I even went as far as having them clean the vans they were driving the fighters around in. Edwin ended up getting hospitalized. Dana went as far as to say I saved the season, and now the UFC watches out for it. It ended up being a great season, with Matt Serra going on to defeat

GSP for the UFC welterweight title in a dramatic upset. It often goes overlooked, but probably the most common and dangerous skin infection I have seen is staph."

## RINGWORM

Ringworm is perhaps the most well-known skin infection for grapplers and wrestlers. Ringworm is not caused by a virus (herpes) or a bacteria (staph/impetigo). Instead, ringworm is caused by a fungal infection. The proper name for ringworm is tinea corporis, but since the infection often leads to a red, scaly, ring-shaped lesion with a clear center, the name ringworm took hold. Like the other skin infections presented in this chapter, ringworm can be transmitted by skin-to-skin contact and can develop in many different areas of the body. Again, proper hygiene is important and all rashes should be covered to prevent spread. Anti-fungal medications can also be prescribed to battle this condition.

Sean Sherk advises looking out for yourself and your training partners. "I had ringworm two or three times. There have been a lot of guys at the gym that come in with that. I don't know why guys show up with that and train and won't tell you. If you have an infection, just get out of there. Train another day."

Like many fighters, grappling coach Dean Lister has seen ringworm and has some tips on avoiding it. "If you are the 1% that has never had a skin infection, then congratulations. For the rest of us, one of the simplest tricks to minimize the chances of getting an infection is to wear a shirt in training and, most importantly, take a shower within 15 minutes of getting off the mat. If you do get something like ringworm, there are appropriate creams you can use to get rid of it."

With all of these infections, prevention and proper hygiene are of utmost importance. According to UFC Hall of Famer Dan Severn, "Ringworm, impetigo, I have had it all. Someone has to bring it in. Personal hygiene is very important. You need to shower right after practice is over. Make sure to clean every piece of equipment, including all floor mats, wall mats, heavy bags, and gloves. And make sure those guys that bring their own equipment also regularly clean it. I make my athletes leave their shoes at the door and off the mats." Frank Shamrock prefers to keep things simple when it comes to keeping equipment clean: "I don't wear a gi. It's one less thing to clean and harbor bacteria."

## CHAPTER 9

# WEIGHT-CUTTING, PEDS, AND TRT

## WEIGHT-CUTTING

One of the most significant health issues currently facing the sport of MMA is weight-cutting. Fighters have been known to cut up to 20 pounds for a weigh-in merely a day or two before their fight. Of course, weigh-ins have been a standard for combat sports for generations, but there is a significant difference between a steady and controlled weight-cut and losing weight at the last minute only to then put it all back on to have an advantage over your opponent.

Some fighters seem to have no problem making weight, while others struggle. Weigh-ins can be daunting, and not making weight could make the difference between a chance in the UFC and not making rent. It is not unheard of for fighters to dehydrate themselves to the point of needing intravenous fluids right after the weigh-in. The crazy thing is, many bouts are between two fighters who weighed in at the same weight class but then fight the next night, both at the same weight — one weight class above the one they weighed in at! As many fighters can tell you, a drastic or "hard" weight-cut can sometimes lead to a suboptimal performance when the actual bout begins.

Some weight-loss methods can prove detrimental to a fighter's health. The most simple but dangerous weight-cutting practice is starvation or fasting. Significant starvation can cause your body to enter a state of emergency as it struggles to break down its own fat, and if necessary, muscle storages, leading to high levels of dangerous substances in the blood such as lactate and ketones.

Another unhealthy method of weight loss is the use of diet pills or laxatives. Many diet pills contain substances that supposedly increase your body's metabolism, but in reality your body will experience an increased heart rate and/or high blood pressure, possibly even to dangerous levels. In addition, laxatives can lead to dehydration from excessive water loss and not allow the body to absorb the nutrients it needs before the food is pushed through the body. Furthermore, some of the diet pills and laxatives contain ingredients that are banned by national and international sports organizations and could lead to a suspension and fine if detected.

Dehydration is a result of more fluid being expelled than consumed. When fighters sweat but don't drink any liquids, they will lose weight quickly, but this is a very dangerous practice. Dehydration may lead to electrolyte imbalances that can have serious health consequences. In addition, practices such as working out in garbage bags or saunas can cause your body to overheat and your blood pressure and heart rate to skyrocket, preventing your body from naturally keeping itself under control.

When your organs don't see enough fluid or when electrolyte imbalances occur, the organs can begin to fail. The two-time Olympic wrestler Daniel Cormier had a scary experience during the 2008 Beijing Games. As is customary with almost all elite-level wrestlers, Cormier was cutting water weight. However, due to his fluid loss, his kidneys began to fail, forcing him to withdraw from the competition. Another UFC veteran, Marcus Davis, has told the story of when he left the UFC and fought for Canada's MFC at 155 pounds. Davis said the cut "nearly killed him," leaving him unable to speak at the weigh-ins because his throat was so coarse from dehydration, and also unable to use the bathroom for several days. And yet a third story circulating the internet is that Rory Markham cut weight so much that his body cramped severely enough to collapse a lung. It's clear there is a problem out there with dangerous weight-cutting techniques and regulation.

What is needed in the sport of MMA is an overall governing body. Unfortunately, the way the system runs now is that each state has its own commission that oversees contests. And even then, fighters can fight on Native American soil and not become subject to state regulations. Many of us in the medical community are trying to find a solution to these issues. In addition, commissions are looking at ways to limit weight-cutting and gain by re-weighing fighters before bouts or limiting the weight classes they can cut down to based on their hydration levels. However, we cannot do it alone. We need the help of the MMA community to identify and solve problems as the sport grows. We also need to discourage the unsafe practices that are out there through education and proper training. There are some good resources available at the NCAA and USA Wrestling websites, as well as some of the state athletic comissions. In addition, you should plan how much you can cut by seeing a certified athletic trainer who can measure your hydration status and body composition and use that information to plan out a safe and healthy weight-cut plan.

As a general guideline, the NCAA promotes the 1.5% rule among its collegiate wrestlers. The 1.5% per week rule states that you should lose no more than 1.5% of your body weight a week. So, a 165-pound athlete should not lose more than two and a half pounds (1.5%) per week. Make sure to recalculate the 1.5% each week. By following this, a 177-pound athlete would safely be at middleweight (170 pounds) after 3 weeks. This rule is in place to minimize the degree of dehydration that results from losing too much body water. Dehydration of even 1% of your body weight decreases your body's endurance and physical performance. Losing weight is best done by creating a calorie deficit of 500 to 1,000 calories per day both by increasing physical activity and decreasing food intake. This approach results in slower weight loss but a greater likelihood that the weight lost will be primarily from fat, not water or muscle. Some basic strategies to help you reach your weight goal are: set a reasonable goal and avoid trying to make a weight class that is not realistic or safe for your body; plan ahead to know where your weight needs to be and consider the time you need to get there safely; adequately fuel your body all day — by skipping meals during the day and eating a lot at night you may encourage storage of body fat and use of lean tissue for energy.

## PEDS AND TRT

Another controversial issue in MMA, and in all sports, is the use of performance enhancing drugs (PEDs). PEDs have no place in professional sports, and fighters who abuse them should be punished. A recent topic of controversy has been the use of synthetic testosterone for therapeutic use. The chemical signaling pathway of the body is called the endocrine system and it is a very complex system, interweaving several different parts of the body secreting several different types of hormones, or chemical signals. When the testosterone level in the blood is low, sometimes referred to as low "T," the hypothalamus in the brain releases gonadotropin-releasing hormone (GnRH), which triggers cells in the front of the pituitary gland, located at the base of the brain. The pituitary gland then releases luteinizing hormone (LH) and follicle-stimulating hormone (FSH). These two hormones then act on the testes. The LH triggers the testes to produce testosterone. Then, when the amount of testosterone in the body reaches an acceptable level, the hypothalamus senses this and stops releasing GnRH. This intricate balance of production and inhibition can be disrupted anywhere along the way, either by decreasing the production of a specific hormone or preventing the necessary feedback sensors from knowing how much hormone is circulating in the blood.

While testosterone replacement therapy is not approved for athletic competition, some athletes are given therapeutic exemptions, because they have documented low levels of testosterone. There is a long laundry list of causes of low testosterone, and many are applicable to MMA fighters and other athletes. Some include anabolic steroid abuse, painkiller abuse, head trauma, and weight-cutting. Of these, head trauma, and weight-cutting are the most controversial, because, ostensibly the fighter hasn't done anything wrong other than prepare for his match and absorb physical punishment.

The most plausible and researched cause for hypogonadism (when the body can't produce normal amounts of testosterone), according to studies published in fairly reputable journals, seems to be pituitary dysfunction after head trauma. Whether MMA athletes receive head trauma severe enough to cause this remains a question. Low testosterone from weight-cutting or weight loss is less researched, and even those studies that have looked at it don't show a direct causation between weight loss and low testosterone levels. For example, one study of wrestlers competing in several bouts during a single-day tournament showed that while testosterone levels do decline below normal from the beginning of the tournament to the end, shortly after the matches, the testosterone levels actually spike above normal.[3] In addition, there is a lot more going on during a tournament than simply weight loss. Thus, it's hard to connect weight loss to low levels of testosterone.

In the general population, the rate of hypogonadism tends to be a low 2%, and the vast majority of these people aren't elite athletes. However, it seems that the percentage of MMA fighters asking for or using TRT is much higher than the expected 2% of the population. Some people point to steroid abuse or head trauma as specific causes, which may be more prevalent in the MMA population and, therefore, it's not surprising to see high levels of athletes requiring TRT. Others see the use of TRT simply as an attempt to cheat the system. Certainly, if a fighter has low testosterone due to steroid abuse, giving him TRT after that may seem to be compounding the athlete's abuse of PEDs. As a result, California and Nevada currently no longer allow for therapeutic use exemptions (TUEs) for TRT, and it is likely many states who wish to discourage using TRT as a PED will follow suit.

---

3 "Physiological and performance adaptations of elite Greco-Roman wrestlers during a one-day tournament." *Eur J Appl Physiol.* 2011 Jul; 111(7): 1421–36. doi: 10.1007/s00421-010-1761-7. Epub 2010 Dec 16. Barbas I, Fatouros IG, Douroudos II, Chatzinikolaou A, Michailidis Y, Draganidis D, Jamurtas AZ, Nikolaidis MG, Parotsidis C, Theodorou AA, Katrabasas I, Margonis K, Papassotiriou I, Taxildaris K.

When it comes to supplements, science often takes a back seat to opinion or personal experience. The vast majority of supplements fighters and other athletes use have never been shown to speed up recovery or improve performance by validated scientific studies. That is not to say they don't help; there is just no sound scientific data to justify using them. That being said, if a fighter stays smart and researches what he or she is putting into his or her body, they can try to find an advantage and lower the risk of hurting themselves. Discussing all of your supplements with your doctor is very important, as some of them may interact with each other or affect the way medications work. In addition, the supplement industry is not tightly regulated, and you may not know what substances are actually in what you're taking. There are some services available to the athlete that will actually test your supplements to make sure there are no harmful or banned substances in them.

## CHAPTER 10

# INJURY PREVENTION: THE KEY LESSONS

Throughout my interviews and conversations with the fighters and trainers featured in this book, several themes were repeated. This should attest to the importance of these lessons in injury prevention. While many of these rules may seem obvious or simple, the actual application of these rules to MMA training are either overlooked or not deeply understood by the fighter and his team. Here we will explore them with some of MMA's top talent. The top five most repeated principles of injury prevention are:

1. Choose the right camp and surround yourself with a good team.
2. Use proper equipment in all aspects of training.
3. Listen to your body (not your ego) and adapt.
4. Avoid overtraining.
5. Train smarter, not harder.

## CHOOSE THE RIGHT CAMP AND
## SURROUND YOURSELF WITH A GOOD TEAM

Surrounding yourself with a good team is often a disregarded part of injury prevention, especially in mixed martial arts. Professional athletes in more mainstream sports are usually part of a large organization that includes doctors, certified athletic trainers, physical therapists, massage therapists, strength and conditioning coaches, and more. The MMA athlete is often limited to who his gym has hired. They may be working with the best striking coaches or grappling coaches in the area, but they may not be surrounded with people who are specifically trained in injury prevention and treatment. Finding a training team that is knowledgeable and experienced is important in fostering your growth as an athlete. Legendary UFC champion Randy Couture has some advice for newer fighters: "Younger guys are restless and tend to jump around from camp to camp even while they're preparing for a specific fight. Having continuity in the training environment is very important to achieving a peak performance and measuring your progress in a sport where experience is very valuable."

However, you should branch out and avoid limiting yourself to the teachings of just one camp. And while the process of finding a good camp should be continuous and updated as necessary, you should always have a core training family to return to. As Brandon Vera, a veteran of the UFC and ONE FC, recommends, "Finding good training partners and coaches will always be an ongoing journey for you, because you should never want to stop learning. You should be going to other gyms, learning new things, sharing new things, and bringing them back to your home gym. There are a lot of coaches/training partners with good intentions, but they are not necessarily good training partners. Some camps are all about being tough, some are all about being technical, some are more of a stand-up school, and the list goes on and on. So you can still go out and learn, but choose the training partners you return home to carefully. These people will sweat with you, bleed with you, cry and laugh with you.

So it has to be a good vibe and a good fit. They become your family, so you can go out and learn, but always bring this knowledge back home to your family."

Carlos Condit finds that not all camps fit all fighters, and you need to find a camp that works for you and promotes your progress and style. "Where I train, at Jackson's MMA, there are a lot of great guys, but it's not super structured. You have to be self-motivated, which I am. But a lot of guys can get lost in the shuffle. There is no one telling you when to show up for practice. Some guys need more encouragement. You need to find what type of camp works for you."

You need to surround yourself not only with good coaches, but also with safe, reliable training partners. It takes a team to build a champion. Nate "Rock" Quarry, a UFC and MMA veteran, as well as co-host of the TV show *MMA Uncensored Live*, sees egos in training partners as a potential source of injury. "The fight game, by its very nature, is filled with egos. Your training partner may want to hit you just a little harder than you hit him. He may never let you work to get back on top when he gets the better of you. He could be the legendary 'Club Pro' or 'Focus Mitt Superstar.' Those are the guys that, while they never fight professionally at a high level, have to make sure all the athletes in the gym know how good they are. And they do that by refusing to 'flow.'

"With a good partner, you develop the 'flow' in training. You train each other and both get better as a result. For example, if he's working on his head movement to avoid getting hit so much, I'll slow down my punches, let him see them coming so he develops the necessary skill to avoid them. And, shockingly enough, he gets better and gives me a better partner to train with so we both win. I see it all the time in sparring sessions, a live version of Rock 'em Sock 'em Robots. And every time I see that happening all I can think to myself is, 'Man, I'm glad I know I'm tough so I don't have to prove it every day in the gym.'"

Quarry goes on to say, "Make sure you find a good camp and a great coach. A coach who cares about your success and safety — not just the winning record of his gym. Train with partners that understand the fight isn't in the gym. The fight is in the cage. The gym is where you prepare for it. Every champion is built. They are an amalgam of their coaches and training partners. They are standing on the shoulders of giants who helped them reach new heights. Or, if you aren't paying attention, those coaches and training partners could be tearing down the house you built, brick by brick. Perhaps maliciously, perhaps out of ignorance. Either way the end result is the same: a busted career and, most likely, a busted body."

Don Frye and Mark Coleman first met at *UFC 10*. Since that time, these two MMA pioneers have spread the same two key pieces of advice to new fighters. Don Frye remarks, "My advice to new guys is two things: one, take the time to stretch, and two, find a good team. Fortunately, my career was 13–15 years long, but I didn't have the patience to stretch. If I did, I could have stolen a couple more years. As for number two: surround yourself with quality, professional people. That's really the first thing you should do. Start with a trainer who knows what he is doing and doesn't put you in risky situations. And your sparring partners need to know they are just sparring partners. In our camps, guys would come in fighting like they were there to win the world title, and we were quick to kick them out."

Mark Coleman almost echoes what his fellow MMA pioneer advises. "What I never did when I was younger, but now I know better, is stretch. You have to stretch to protect yourself. Do yoga or something similar. Being flexible can help you prevent injuries. In the weight room I was old school, just ripping out heavy weights. I just assumed the stronger guy wins. But now I am older and wiser and stress technique and stretching. I do yoga. As for what you and your team do in practice, when you train, save all the dangerous moves for the cage. Make sure you and your partners are on the same page. You are there as a team to help each other out. Injuries can ruin your career. You need to simulate the fight, but don't do dangerous moves that can end your or your partner's career."

Being a good training partner is a give-and-take relationship, so that both of you can improve the skills you'll need for your next fight. Josh Barnett, an MMA veteran and the youngest UFC Heavyweight Champion in UFC history, understands that fighters need to "build a relationship with your training partner and let them know if you do beat them up in training, you won't go out on the internet and talk trash. Both of you need to know that the fighter needs to focus on his opponent and what they bring to the fight. So, if they need a southpaw, and you are a southpaw, you will be there for him. If your opponent is orthodox, understand they may need someone else. They also need to remember to help focus on my improvement by letting me lead. Trust that I am not looking to hurt you in training. I want you to come back tomorrow or next week. And I will do the same. Instead of looking to kick your butt while you are training, I will give you the opportunity to see what you need to improve on and [will let you] use me to work on that."

MMA veteran and Olympic silver-medalist wrestler Matt Lindland knows what it takes to make a great team. "The 2000 Olympic wrestling team was one of the greatest teams I was ever a part of. It's not that we didn't have problems, because we had plenty, but what made the team so great was we had such great team members. What is it that makes a great teammate? Great teammates are finishers. Great teammates hold themselves and their teammates accountable. They get the job done. They finish what they start. They keep their word. When they say they will meet you for an extra conditioning workout, they show up on time ready to go.

"Great teammates anticipate, understand what needs to be done next, and look for ways to step up and help the team. One of my teammates at the Olympic training center did not make the Olympic squad but was one of the most valuable teammates we brought with us to Sydney. This man got an apartment right next to the wrestling venue, so we had a place to rest in between rounds. No one asked him to do it, he just showed up and took care of it. Little things like this can make such an impact. Finally, great teammates are humble. Pride comes before a fall, and for teams the same holds true. A teammate should always be pulling others up to their level and never tearing others down. They never criticize the leadership or their teammates, especially in public."

MMA coach Renzo Gracie has advice for fighters looking for a good camp. Make sure the guys you train with leave you feeling comfortable knowing that they aren't going to try and hurt you or test you too much. "You need to pick guys you are comfortable with. I remember how guys would come from all over the world to spar with Georges St-Pierre, so he would always have to give it 100%. It's tiring. He looked forward to coming to me to relax and just train jiu-jitsu. You can't take away a guy's comfort zone. He needs to know his training partners are not there to hurt him. I once saw GSP train for seven different rounds with seven different guys. This is too demanding. You can't relax. You can't grow. George told me he looked forward to retiring so he could just relax and do jiu-jitsu. You don't want to have to kill a lion every day. You want to feel comfortable with the guys around you."

Dan Severn notes, "I set up most of my workouts and training camps myself. I just had good people that were around me and we had safe camps, too. When you hear or you read about all these upcoming cards, how people are getting hurt and the change of opponents or scratching of matches, a lot of it, I truly believe, can be prevented by running a proper training camp. There's no way that you can train 100% and still have workout partners. Or your workout partners will get so sick of becoming punching bags for you that, because they're human beings, they'll want to take it back out on you. It's a give-and-take relationship."

EDUCATE YOURSELF IN THE PROCESS

Josh Barnett has long realized the importance of surrounding yourself with reliable and educated people. "The biggest difference between [MMA] and more mainstream sports is the money they have at their disposal. Each football team spends hundreds of millions of dollars on players every year. No one fighter will ever equal that. You are only one athlete. That being said, you don't need an entire NFL staff. But if you want care and training at the highest level, you will need to spend money. If you want the highest level of knowledge, you need to invest in yourself. In Japan, I used to hire Stitch to come out with me to do my cuts and wrap my hands. Folks would see him around and wanted his expertise, but they would have to pay for his services. While many guys hired him, other guys thought the meager amount of a couple of hundred dollars was not worth the investment of a world-class hand wrapper and cutman. Unfortunately that's the mentality of many fighters in MMA — to get more for less. But if you work with guys in a more direct manner and form a relationship, like I did with Stitch, you will not only be around experts, but you will also learn from them. He taught me to wrap hands properly. If I wanted to, he could teach me how to treat cuts. You are responsible for you at the end of the day."

## USE PROPER EQUIPMENT

Wearing and using proper equipment and protection is paramount. Whether it's correctly applied hand wraps, headgear, or even clean mats, proper equipment can help prevent a lot of injuries. Headgear should be worn any time there is a chance of getting a head-butt, even if you aren't practicing striking. If you are practicing striking, you should be using heavier gloves (around 16oz) for your hands and padding your shins and elbows. Save the MMA gloves for grappling and technical work. Vaseline and a well-fitting mouthguard should also be in your equipment bag. The gym you are training at should use permanent or roll-out mats instead of puzzle mats. For Frank Shamrock, you can never protect yourself too much. "If you are going full contact, pad every surface. Either you train in a strictly technical way or you have contact. At the end of my career I had a pad on every square inch of my body. I even use a lubricant on the face and other bony surfaces to prevent injury."

Pat Miletich is the founder of Miletich Fighting Systems, which has spawned UFC champions Matt Hughes, Tim Sylvia, Jens Pulver, and Robbie Lawler. He also makes sure his fighters are using the correct equipment for sparring. "I am a heavy believer in padding our guys up fully. When our guys spar full-contact, we never use MMA gloves. We use 16 oz gloves, headgear, and shin pads so they can train at fight-speed. Guys training striking with MMA gloves develop bad habits like not hitting fully and leaning back to avoid fingers coming into eyes. I like using MMA gloves more for technique in the mornings, but then we use full boxing gloves at night for striking practice."

However, just wearing gear isn't always enough — you have to make sure it's the right gear and that it's doing its intended job. "When you spar," Bas Rutten says, "pay attention to your protecting gear. If it gets old, buy new gear! Take your time to 'pack yourself up.' You don't want to go into an MMA fight with an injury from training." And since one cut can derail your entire training camp, elite trainer Mark DellaGrotte makes sure all of his fighters use headgear. "I have seen a lot of guys get a big cut or even a broken orbital from a knee to the face. I understand a lot of guys don't like to wear headgear because it's cumbersome and it's hard to grapple with and get out of chokes with. But as the fight gets closer, you need to make sure you stay healthy enough to get to the fight in top shape. The last thing anyone wants to do, including the fighters and the promoters, is to have to cancel a fight because a guy gets hurt. As the fight gets closer, all my guys are using headgear and large boxing gloves."

Gilbert Melendez always wears protective gear, but adjusts it based on what type of training he is doing. "Anytime I am punching, I am wrapping my hands. I wrap them with cloth hand wrap and then tape over the top of the wrap. Anytime I am sparring I have headgear, 16 oz gloves, and the thickest pads, not just MMA pads. I use elbow and knee pads and always wear a cup. For strictly MMA sparring, I may go with thinner pads. And every day, I throw on Vaseline, even if it's on strictly jiu-jitsu or wrestling days."

Besides padding, mouthguards are an important part of training. Andy Foster, former MMA fighter and CSAC commissioner, calls his mouthpiece "the most personal piece of equipment" he owns. No matter where he was or who he was fighting, he had his mouthpiece with him. Make sure to use a mouthguard that fits your mouth. There are boil and bite models as well as professionally made mouthguards custom fit by dentists. In addition, there are now dual-arch mouthguards that cover both the upper and lower teeth. Foster prefers a fitted, dual-arch mouthguard. There is some thought that this dual-arch technology may help limit the amount of trauma the brain receives by absorbing and distributing some of the impact of a jaw punch.

## LISTEN TO YOUR BODY (NOT YOUR EGO) AND ADAPT

The next three keys to injury prevention work in unison. Following the principle of listening to your body and adapting keeps you out of dangerous situations and allows you to still progress in training or in a fight. You can then focus on structuring your training regimen appropriately with the final two principles: ensuring you don't overtrain and training smarter, not harder. Step one in listening to your body is to leave your ego at the door. Sure, tough guys enter the world of mixed martial arts, but there is a difference between being tough and being ignorant. Don't push your body until it breaks down. Don't refuse to tap or give up a takedown during training.

If you aren't performing at your normal level of training, focus on something else rather than putting yourself at injury risk. Good coaches also recognize this and need to protect fighters from themselves and their egos, especially if they are tired and underperforming. When that happens, the fighter and his training partners are at risk for injury. And if an injury does occur or something is painful, listen to your body. Back off on the things that hurt and focus on other areas of your game strategy. That is the adaptation portion of the principle. You must adapt to the situation at hand. Like Bruce Lee, you need to "be like water." You may end up becoming a more well-rounded fighter in the process.

UFC champion Demetrious Johnson knows his body can't handle going hard doing the same routine all the time. "This is the only body I have for my career. Be smart. A guy has to make sure he doesn't get hurt but is also ready for a fight. I know my body better than my coach Matt Hume. I talk to him. You have to communicate with your coach. I let him know what's hurting. We then try alternatives to push my body in other ways. What works for me as a fighter, works for my body."

## HOW TO BE A GOOD COACH

When training top-level fighters, a coach has to pay attention to a fighter's body — pushing him to his limit, but encouraging him to rest before he gets injured. It's not always enough to just listen to a fighter, because they won't always vocalize how they're feeling or when something hurts. Sometimes a coach has to be more intuitive and has to know what their fighter needs before the fighter knows. This can mean altering the game plan, even on fight night. Pat Miletich, coach to Tim Sylvia and Robbie Lawler, recalls having to train Jens Pulver for an upcoming fight while avoiding further injury to Jens's back. "Jens Pulver had hurt his back going into a fight against John Lewis, a strong grappler. Jens is an All-American wrestler who could match Lewis on the ground, but Jens is also a solid boxer. From watching John, I knew he would throw a southpaw jab and would drop his hand. By focusing on out-striking Lewis rather than out-wrestling him, we could spare Jens having to stress his back on the ground. In the fight, Lewis threw the jab, and Jens threw a counter that missed. But the second time the window opened, Jens shattered Lewis's jaw. Again, if there is an injury, we have to work around it. We have to do that a lot in the sport. It comes down to keeping fighters safe and still helping them win.

"As a coach or fighter, you also have to change your practice plans too. Often we would have running practice and also drill takedowns in the same session. Takedowns are the most physical aspect of the sport. Guys are trying to post and stop a takedown, but this can lead to injury if the guys are tired. In fact, I think a lot of guys need to learn the fundamentals of wrestling. They need to learn how to land.

I try to keep guys fresh. When I saw guys starting to land wrong or they got tired, I stopped it and we took a break. Then we changed the practice to ground fighting. As a coach it's important to make sure your fighter is practicing safely."

Renzo Gracie recalls a story from his grandfather, which he applies to the fighters in his camp. "A common mistake coaches make is driving guys too hard. I remember hearing about how my grandfather had trained a farm rooster into a fighting rooster. He could get the rooster to fight for 20 minutes. I asked how he did it. He told me he would have the rooster fight until he got tired but wouldn't let him get hurt by the big fighting roosters. He would pull him back before he got hurt. You have to do the same with your fighters. Otherwise if he gets hurt or trains too hard, he will think about that and it will stick with him. This separates a good coach from an ordinary one."

Greg Nelson, another legendary MMA trainer of UFC champions Sean Sherk and Brock Lesnar, reiterates these sentiments. "Fighters have to listen to their bodies and trainers have to listen to their fighters. If a fighter has all the ingredients to be a champion, he probably won't want to appear weak and will always want to push hard. It is up to the trainer to design a program that will allow the fighter to progressively develop their conditioning and skill level so that they peak on competition day. Then they need to rest, recover, and reevaluate their performance."

## WORKING AROUND INJURIES

If you do have an injury, you need to learn to work around it. Don't go home and sit on the couch and don't push through the pain just to keep doing your typical, unadjusted routine. Pat Miletich recalls, "Over a 20-year period of coaching guys, I learned to work around injuries. Many fighters, including myself, often hurt their dominant striking hand. I saw that as an opportunity to work on the lead hand. I saw injuries as a blessing in disguise. When I injured my right shoulder, I still managed to fight three times professionally, because

I controlled the fight with my left hand. I even focused on using my hand for other activities. For example, I practiced shooting free throws with my left hand."

The last few days before fight night require considerable discipline on the part of the fighter and his training camp. Nerves are running high and every minute not spent training feels like an opportunity for an opponent to gain an advantage. Dean Lister understands this and can relate to his fellow fighters, but he knows listening to his ego can lead to injury. "As fighters, we all think that the extra little bit we do will help. I can't tell you how many fighters I've known, me included, that thought the last day of hard sparring four days before the fight would give me an edge. But instead, it can often result in injury. It's like a curse. I call it the 'last week curse.' Be careful what you do in training camp the days leading up to a fight and always be careful who you train with before a fight."

## AVOID OVERTRAINING

Since MMA has no traditional "off-season," it is important to maintain a steady, healthy level of fitness year round, but it's also imperative that you don't burn yourself out when it comes to training for a fight. Legendary two-weight-class UFC champion Randy Couture offers his advice on injury prevention: "The biggest issue I see in MMA injuries is that fighters' fitness levels wax and wane between competition. MMA is obviously an intense contact sport, so accidents and injuries are going to happen no matter what. I notice younger fighters especially lay off training until they have a fight signed, and then make the difficult climb back into top fight shape, putting their bodies under more than usual physical stress. It's this up and down in fitness where I see the majority of more serious injuries occur. These injuries are usually more serious and are the type that affect your athleticism and life in the long term. They can be avoided by maintaining a higher level of fitness activity between fights. This stresses your body less severely and allows for the achievement of peak competition fitness with less risk of fatigue-based injuries. Make fitness a lifestyle and train with a team you know and trust that has your best interest and athletic development at heart. Listen to your body. Nobody knows it better than you do."

Once you have signed up for a fight and begun your training camp, entering with a base-level of fitness will help prevent early-camp injuries. Then, as you enter into deeper parts of your camp, it's important not to overtrain. Nate Quarry has felt the sharp edge of overtraining. "One time, I signed for a big fight months in advance. Since I knew my opponent was tough, I really kicked my training into overdrive. Some days training three times a day! And of course, to me, every workout was the most important workout of the day, so I trained to exhaustion at each of the three sessions. And when fight week came, I stepped on the scale Friday afternoon and made weight easily, then spent the next five hours vomiting violently with a 102 degree fever. I'd overtrained. Of course I fought the next day. When fighting is how you feed your family, sometimes you have to make unwise decisions. And I did my best. I gave it my all. And I lost in the first round. That was my ego getting the better of me. As fighters and athletes, the easy thing for us is to work. The easy thing is to show people how tough we are. The hardest thing is to rest when we need it. To ice down our sore shoulders. To get regular massages. To get stretched out. To warm up properly. I needed a head coach that could save me from myself. The best coaches are scheduling the workouts and, sometimes more importantly, the much needed rest."

As a coach and fighter, Josh Barnett understands that a coach that has a strong relationship with their athlete can help encourage the fighter to take a step back during training, and the fighter will trust that it's the right decision. "[Fighters] might complain, but they listen, because we develop trust in our relationship. And if I am wrong, I admit it and we make adjustments because we are a team. As a coach, my word is not law, but I am accountable for what I tell my athletes and helping them accomplish what they want. If they want to be a world champion, I expect world champion output. That's how I get them to listen. I provide an example of someone who follows through on their word, and I understand that they are all individuals, not just carbon copies. They each have different physical capabilities and different performance outputs.

"As an athlete you need to just sit back and breathe. Be honest with yourself. You know when you are doing enough. If you aren't, you can't just do more to make up for it. When you hit overtraining, you don't sleep through the night. You are on edge. Your energy levels fall in training and you constantly feel tired, like you're underwater — you can't push harder through that. You need to step back and shorten your workout — keep moving and stay limber, but also give yourself some time to rest. Get a massage and go to a spa. Whenever I hear interviews, I always listen to athletes telling everyone how many hours a day they are training, as if that's the benchmark of their performance. I say, if you are training eight hours a day, then you aren't trying hard enough. With me and my athletes, two to three hours a day is enough."

Renzo Gracie is not only a veteran MMA fighter and pioneer, but also a top-level coach. As a coach it's his responsibility to help his fighters avoid overtraining. "You see the most overtraining in the most insecure athletes. They worry too much about the fight and train too much. As a coach, you have to look at the fighter's personality. Follow and examine what he does on a daily basis. For example, with Frankie Edgar, we would just do positions for two hours. He would train in the morning and then come to me and then go train again after lunch. It was my job during my time with him to calm him down and work on technique. I would just push him mentally. I had to make it fun and make him relaxed. He had to enjoy being there. Then he would be fresh for his training. One of the main reasons you see us sitting down in a circle, smiling, is because we talk, we crack jokes. This takes their mind away from their worries, even the day before the fight. This helps them perform better."

It is the balance between maintaining a good year-round level of fitness and avoiding overtraining that is a key to being a successful athlete and fighter, and also avoiding injuries. As only "El Guapo" Bas Rutten can describe it: "The guys who don't run out of gas, the ones that shine, like Benson Henderson, Frankie Edgar, Cain Velasquez, etc., those guys train really, really hard and know how to train, so they take rest. I overtrained myself a long time ago. I was three months out of commission. At the time, I had only 4% body fat. I was very dumb. Nobody told me I needed rest in order to get stronger. So I trained seven days a week, two times a day, full-out. Needless to say, I collapsed one day. After that, I saw what happened when I took a day off. I got even stronger, I was amazed. Nowadays everybody knows what to eat and how much to rest. I was stupid, even training on beer, steak, and pizza!"

Gilbert Melendez understands that fighters need a certain amount of time to train for a fight. But if you are overtraining or getting too tired, you need to take some time off. A remedy to take time off, but still have the same number of strong training days under your belt when you step in the cage? Extend your training camp a little. "During training camp, listen to your body. Have your map of how you are going to approach training camp. But if you plan on doing some hard wrestling or hard striking and are feeling overtrained, pull back and focus on light training or technique. You can work on just footwork. As a fighter, that light day is tough, and if you are anxious about your upcoming fight, you may feel you need to play catch-up. You will find yourself at a crossroads in your camp. Maybe you need to have a longer camp. Instead of an eight-week camp, do a 10-week camp, and take two to three more days off. You still get the same training and get more days off. Also being in good cardio shape makes you feel better about taking some time off and not losing anything."

It can also help to take a scientific approach to ensure you are training at an appropriate intensity and to help you track what you are doing and how much you are improving. As Carlos Newton suggests, "A key to avoid overtraining is record keeping. Your coach must keep data on what you are doing — for every day and for every activity. When I did that, I didn't overtrain. It also helps navigate psychologically through the ups and downs of training. I have had training stretches where I felt I needed to push harder and wasn't getting enough out of the workout, and my trainer could look at the data and see I was doing eight minutes per circuit where last week I was doing nine minutes. With data, you can see if your performance has improved, even if you feel it hasn't. Work-wise you are stronger or faster, but it becomes psychological. Record keeping helps to set goals, but also motivates without overtraining. You don't need to train based solely on gut feeling. Keep the gut feelings for the fight in the cage."

No fighter is the same and no fighter has the same goals or the same baseline fitness level. Therefore, it's up to you and your coaches to find the fitness regimen that's right for you, instead of mimicking someone else's that may have been successful for them. Ray Longo, trainer to both UFC champions Chris Weidman and Matt Serra, is a big proponent of individualizing his training camps to make sure his guys stay healthy. "Everything we do is on an individual basis. The goal is to get the guy to the fight as healthy as possible. Some of our training camps are as short as five weeks, depending on the guy. You have to experiment and you have to research. Don't take everything you hear as gospel. Research what you hear and what you read. I teach my guys I don't have all the answers, but we will work together to get you where you need to be as safely as we can with a good training camp." Randy Couture tells his guys to look out for signs of overtraining. "Increased insomnia or elevated resting heartrate are indicators of physical overtraining."

CROSS-TRAINING AND ACTIVE DAYS OF REST

Pat Miletich notes, "Most winners in my camp had a strong work ethic. But we also took a day off and focused on cross-training. We might go do one hour of swimming." Dan Severn recalls, "I think overtraining is more of an American trait. Through my career spanning the globe, I was exposed to international training where I have seen wrestlers actually go out and play soccer for one hour rather than spend the day in the gym. They are out there running and having fun and at the same time, actually doing some cross-training. I call it 'active rest.' You can go play basketball or even just take a hike. As an NCAA wrestling coach, I will take guys to the sand volleyball court on campus to run barefoot, practice falling on the sand, and feel what it's like to train on sand. It's a fun alternative way to keep training. We have even gone to the beach and practiced throwing each other in the water."

Like Dan Severn, UFC heavyweight and Brazilian Jiu-Jitsu World Champion Jeff Monson has some strategies to avoid overtraining while still working your body. "Unfortunately, I learned the hard way about overtraining. I have always been a hard worker and willing to push through fatigue and pain barriers. However, many times I was guilty of overtraining. I remember having insomnia, losing interest in outside activities, and inevitably injuring myself while training. Along with separating days between maximum effort and more technical practices, I have found that having what I call 'active rest days' are great to incorporate into a training regimen. This involves doing a completely different sport or training than martial arts. For me this means once a week, I will play pick-up basketball at the gym or go swimming. These active-rest-day activities also have an added bonus of working different muscles that I didn't typically use while boxing, grappling, or [doing] other MMA related practices. This has helped me keep mentally and physically fresh. Training hard but taking the time to stay invigorated and adding variety to the training has worked for me."

## KEEPING YOUR MIND IN THE GAME

If you need mental stimulation to get your mind off overtraining, Army Ranger and UFC veteran Tim Kennedy has some advice for you, "It's hard to not overtrain. To step in a cage and not worry about being unprepared is scary. But, I have some tricks to focus on other things: video games, reloading ammo, gun smithing, and working on guns. You need to find something to do where you can focus on working on your mind and not your body." Like Tim Kennedy, UFC

Heavyweight Champion Tim Sylvia also likes to keep his mind and body busy to help avoiding overtraining. "I believe in active rest — doing something where you can run around and keep active, but also letting yourself have a day off. I like to play paintball or go hunting."

If guns aren't your style, Cesar Gracie has another option for you — yoga. "Many years ago, it was all train, train, train. Training helps fighters in a camp settle their nerves, but then they overtrain. You leave the best part of you outside the cage. You need to go into the fight feeling good, not tired. If they have to do an activity, I tell them to do something healthy like yoga. It's a workout but not a training stress. Someone else might like swimming. You should do low impact exercises and know when to take breaks."

## ICE AS A RECOVERY TOOL

Don't forget about ice during recovery periods, especially for reducing inflammation. The ice works to constrict the blood vessels around the muscles and joints to reduce bloodflow, which helps reduce inflammation and soreness. Granted, there are arguments against using ice after workouts because the post-injury inflammation may be beneficial to long-term endurance enhancement, but the majority of college and professional athletic trainers still use it on their athletes and it appears to be doing its job. Frank Shamrock points out, "Ice is a wonderful tool. I learned it doing physical therapy. It helps to calm and rest your body and let it do amazing things." Brandon Vera also feels ice baths are one of the many parts of a healing regimen. "My best advice for injury prevention includes warming up, stretching, listening to your body, and learning the difference between pain and injury. And don't forget an ice bath at least twice a week at the end of training." To further optimize the benefits of ice, you can utilize the principle of contrast by alternating hot and cold. The heat helps to dilate blood vessels, increasing bloodflow to the sore areas, and the cold constricts the muscles and blood vessels. The alternating contrast can help flush out soreness-inducing lactic acid and lead to a quicker recovery.

## TRAIN SMARTER, NOT HARDER

Above all else, the mantra "train smarter, not harder" has emerged as the greatest take-home message. The first generation of stars in mixed martial arts entered uncharted territory. They had no reassurance that the organization they were fighting for would ever have another event, or if they would even be physically able to fight in an event again. Thus, every injury was a barrier to a payday and a barrier to the growth of the sport. As a result, many of the fighters trained and fought through injuries, ignoring medical advice or denying what their bodies were trying to tell them. As a result, their bodies eventually wore down, and many feel the effects on their careers to this day. There is no doubt that these warriors sacrificed themselves for the good of their careers and for the glory of the emerging sport, but today, things are different. MMA athletes do not need to drive their bodies until they break. Greg Nelson's advice on injury prevention and career improvement is that "it is not just about simply training hard, it is about training right." Or as Dan Severn put it, "Young athletes think they are invincible, but sooner or later a car breaks down."

Feared UFC welterweight Matt "The Immortal" Brown stresses the importance of proper training, listening to your body, and maintaining it for the duration of a career. Much like Dan Severn, he sees the body as a car that needs to keep running. "I have been fortunate throughout my career to not have very many debilitating injuries. I attribute this partially to luck but more so to proper training. A lot of trainers think that injuries stem from overtraining. I agree, but I would also argue that they are caused by improper training. A large portion of my daily regimen is focused on prehab: correcting muscular imbalances, creating symmetry, improving mobility, and general strengthening of tendons and ligaments. It's analogous to tightening the nuts and bolts of your car or changing the oil and keeping the chassis lubed. I built a strong vehicle over years of training. Now the important part is fine-tuning the vehicle and performing proper maintenance. I don't get out of shape when I don't have a fight, and this allows time to maintain, build, and fine-tune on a consistent basis. If you have a well maintained vehicle, you can run it harder and more often, which results in better performances in all aspects of your life."

Part of training smarter, not harder is to look beyond just strength, and instead focus on flexibility and functionality. Sure, everyone wants to look good in the gym and when walking into the cage, but don't be one of those guys who spent all their time lifting weights and not enough time training to fight. The key is to balance strength with flexibility. Sean Sherk points to more functional-type training. "Don't grab the heaviest weights in the gym and throw them around. That's how you get hurt. It's a big reason why I got hurt. Over time, I realized I am not in a weightlifting competition. I am a fighter. The key is to train smarter with functional training."

Pat Miletich likes the idea of gravity boots as part of functional training. "They help to strengthen the core and legs. I would do reverse squats, hanging upside, pulling my butt to my heels. I like functional exercises. I would often work out at Turner Halls, which are German-American gymnasiums. They were the original crossfit dating back to the 1900s. We would do kettlebells, Olympic lifts, throwing medicine balls, and pommel horses. It taught me all of the functional fitness I do today."

As has been said multiple times already, a proper warm-up is vital. Warming up the muscles not only prevents injuries, but also helps prepare for hard training; the elevated heart rate increases the blood flow to the muscles and helps relax the joints. Like many veteran fighters, Jeff Monson, an MMA veteran, world-champion grappler, and member of the world class American Top Team, stresses an adequate warm-up before going hard in training. "At American Top Team, we have found that warming up with drilling proper technique at a slow pace that gradually increases over a 30-minute period is an excellent warm-up that solidifies proper technique and prevents injuries."

It's also beneficial to take an introspective approach to your trainings and evaluate your regimen, asking yourself what you are doing and for what reason. Josh Barnett has had much success with this approach. "Whenever something on my body starts hurting, instead of just saying this part of my body hurts and move on, I think about what is actually making it hurt and why, not only for myself but also for my athletes, and I learn from that. Athletes need to get the most they can each day in training, but not by just doing the hardest workout they can do. There are many avenues to consistently improve, whether it's sparring or watching tape. It doesn't matter if you beat up everyone else in the gym or you get beat up. You need to think about what you are doing and always seek to improve your personal MMA journey. The first thing you can do is focus on perfecting technique. That's number one. Then realize that strength and conditioning training doesn't replace fight training. There are many guys who focus on strength and conditioning, but don't have knowledge of fighting. Your strength and conditioning coach is not your fight coach. In fight camps, they are doing ropes, kettlebells, and taxing their body and then sparring hard, and as a result, they can't recover. You exhaust your mental and physical capabilities. You get sluggish in the ring or find yourself in a bad position. There are times when you do need to go hard, but hard training doesn't mean getting suplexed on your head and getting concussions. Going to war every day at your gym may work at your gym, but it may leave a gaping hole in your game outside the gym. The guys I train may get beat in the gym, but that may just be part of where they are in their journey. Look at every workout you do and tailor your camp according to your opponent and where you are on your MMA journey. Don't just participate in mindless training scenarios that don't focus on what you need to improve."

Mixed martial arts is here to stay and is one of the world's fastest growing sports. Athletes are entering the sport in hopes of a long-lived career, just as one would enter more mainstream professional sports. If they are to succeed, they need to learn to train smarter, not harder. Today's mixed martial artist is a multi-dimensional athlete, and as such, fighters and those around them need to bring the athlete to the limits of training, without going over the line into injury territory.

Mark DellaGrotte understands the difference between training hard and training smart. "I see a lot of these younger guys and they try to do too much, too hard. It's a bravado, a 'machismo.' You see these guys in their thirties doing great? It's because they know their body; they know their age, their past injuries, and their limitations. As you get older, you should get wiser. As a sport, we need our fighters to continue to get wiser. To move in the other direction is suicide. When I see a young kid in the gym hitting his shin on one of the poles or support columns, he has to be educated right away that this is not the way to think. If these guys continue in that mentality and in that direction of training, they are moving further away from good health and further away from that title, and maybe even moving towards their demise. A lot of fighters don't realize how hard it is to make it to the big shows like the UFC, but it's even harder to stay there. That doesn't just mean winning fights, it also means staying healthy. A lot of guys have winning records, but can't stay at that level because they can't stay healthy. It starts with good, healthy fitness and awareness. You need to train smartly. It doesn't always have to be bigger and stronger. It should also be smarter."

DellaGrotte continues, "Injury prevention doesn't start when the fighter steps into the Octagon. It begins on day one of training camp. You need to think about everything you are doing from the warm-up onward and make sure you are doing it right. We have made leaps and bounds in fighter preparation and training. When I first started, everyone just went to Thailand and watched what the guys did there. They did a light jog, and that was about it. They didn't have proper conditioning coaches, warm-up, recovery, active rest days, ice baths, or physical therapy. That worked for them, but that doesn't work for today's MMA athlete."

Sometimes it takes an injury to cause a fighter to change his training habits for the better, as was the case for Matt Serra. "The only fight I ever pulled out of was my fight with Matt Hughes. [The fight] was a big deal because we had bad blood. The day I got hurt, I had been purposely training from bad positions since Matt is such a good wrestler. At the end of the session, I was already cooled down, my muscles were tight, and I was ready for the shower. Matt Arroyo, one of my teachers now, asked me to show him a neck crank. I got back on the mat to demonstrate the move and felt my back hurt immediately. I ended up herniating my L4-5 disc. This experience made me change my training habits. I trained smarter after that, always listening to my body. Before the injury, I was going too hard all the time. I was about 34 at the time of my injury. I wasn't in my twenties anymore. I usually would start training by being put in a crucifix hold, then do 20 suplexes, and then go right into the heavy pads. I was getting myself pretty worn out. But as I got older I focused on training smarter, not harder."

Nate Quarry has learned similar lessons in his two decades of fighting. "I've been in and around the fight game for nearly 20 years now. What's the best piece of advice I can give to an up-and-coming fighter? Train smart. That is the best advice I can give you. Take care of your equipment. Don't train injured. Don't overtrain. Don't train with people who don't care about your safety. And don't train under coaches who don't care about your health. Fight for the love of fighting, but you also better treat fighting like a career. And a big part of a successful career is self-preservation. Train smart."

Mixed martial arts is an inherently dangerous sport. Fighters will get hurt, but it is our responsibility as doctors, trainers, coaches, therapists, training partners, and combatants to educate each other on proper training and rehabilitation. Don't just take the advice from someone who you roll with or see at the gym. See a doctor or certified athletic trainer or physical therapist. You don't want to ignore an injury that can easily be treated now, just to have a big surgery down the road. Many fighters are uninsured and therefore don't seek the advice of medical professionals. In the key words from Demetrious Johnson, "Get some insurance if you plan on fighting." And most importantly, educate yourself and remember to train smarter, not harder!

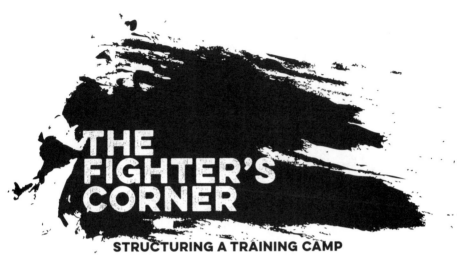

## THE FIGHTER'S CORNER

### STRUCTURING A TRAINING CAMP

WITH GREG NELSON, DEMETRIOUS JOHNSON, AND PAT MILETICH

Proper planning of a training camp is the blueprint for injury prevention and performance improvement that you will follow in order to peak on fight night. Greg Nelson describes how he approaches a fighter's training camp. "A training camp should be eight to 10 weeks maximum. If a fighter is training daily, year round, he should be at about 60% of his optimum fight shape. The training camp is going to be a very directed training camp that is shaped by the opponent that we are preparing to meet. A game plan is devised. Where should the fighter focus the fight? Do they want to keep it standing or pressed up against the cage? Are we fighting a better striker and want to get the fight on the ground or against the cage? Or is our fighter better on the ground but we are fighting a very good takedown blocker or another strong wrestler? There are many factors that come into play. Where are we weak and need to improve and where can we stifle our opponent's attacks?

"I am a big believer in working on as many fight-specific training methods as possible during fight camp. I have recently seen many fighters stress outside conditioning (throwing tires, doing weight training circuits, sprints, etc.) and they come in tired for the actual fight training. If a fighter cannot hit the mitts or Thai Pads like they should, as close to fight pace as possible, or they are fatiguing too fast in live grappling or sparring, they are most likely spending too much of their energy with supplemental training.

"You should have your training sessions broke apart and set up throughout the week. For example, Monday: wake up and run before eating to increase your metabolism and build overall stamina. Know what you are eating and why. Then rest and mentally prepare for the first training session of the week. Monday morning training focuses on takedowns and grappling. Warm up properly and stretch for 30 minutes. Then do striking to takedowns for six 5-minute rounds. Then striking to takedowns again but adding submissions on the ground for 5-minute rounds. Then incorporate MMA-style live grappling with five-minute rounds, starting with striking to takedowns, and once your partner hits the ground it is live. Strikes are controlled, but are placed with enough force to register their potency. At the same time, you are battling for position and submission. After the hard training, focus on building technically sound movements during a fatigued state. Then, take a short water break. A short, sprint-style conditioning session can follow to wrap up the morning session.

"In the afternoon, fighters can do a strength and conditioning circuit. The circuit should be 20–30 minutes, but very intense. It should push the fighters, building what is most needed: muscular endurance, power, speed, agility, or all of the above. Always make sure the fighter is hydrated, has eaten the proper fuel to allow them to push past their perceived limits, and knows what to eat after the session to rest, rebuild, and recover. At this point, having done the hard sessions, it is important to have a drilling session where the fighter focuses 100% on the specific submission or striking skills he wants to build to become a better fighter. This focus on improving weak areas must be part of a fighter's training, if not, he will have holes in his game. This type of day should happen three times a week.

"For sparring sessions, do a variety of striking drills to properly warm up the fighter, physically and mentally. As part of the warmup, do combo for combo, shadow boxing with your partner. Only after the fighters are properly warmed up should you initiate sparring. Sparring rounds start with timing sparring (live but controlled, attempting to build timing over speed), and then gradually build up to full sparring. On the outside, the coach and others should monitor the action, making sure no one is getting hit too much, getting fatigued, losing focus, or allowing their emotions to rule over reason.

"Lastly, there should be a day off for full recovery. It is necessary that the fighter have a game plan that increases in intensity as his conditioning grows. They should always be monitored and the coach should be aware of all of the supplemental conditioning and nutrition that is being done. The fighters must be hydrated, fueled with a proper diet, and getting the necessary sleep."

Some fighters like to do their cardio in the morning and their grappling or sparring at night, keeping at least one or two days off for recovery. A typical training week for Demetrious Johnson begins on Monday morning. "Monday morning I do cardio to get my heart rate up. At night, I do Muay Thai and standup. Tuesday I try to swim a mile and then some brick work and underwater work for recovery. Tuesday night I spar. Wednesday morning is time off and the afternoon is for grappling. Then I take Thursday completely off. Friday, I start up again with cardio and then later in the day pads and MMA/pankration. Saturday I spar again." It's also important to alter your training routine as you get closer to fights. As for when to focus on strength versus speed, Pat Miletich likes to focus more on explosive Olympic lifts 10–12 weeks out from a fight, and as it gets closer to fight day, he concentrates on speed, endurance, and high reps.

# INDEX

Illustrations denoted by *fig.*

A ——————————————

Abbott, Tank, 34, 124
AC separations, 82–83
acetabulum, 101
acromioclavicular (AC) joint, 80
acromioclavicular (AC) separations,
    82–83
acromion, 80, 82 *fig*
active rest, 173–174, 178
    *see also* rest
adductor muscles, 102–103
    adductor brevis, 102 *fig*
    adductor longus, 102 *fig*
    adductor magnus, 102 *fig*
adrenaline for lacerations, 31, 32–33
alcohol, limiting consumption of, 3, 19
Alves, Thiago, 102
American College of Sports Medicine, 2
anterior cruciate ligament (ACL), 48,
    50 *fig*
    grafts, 50–51

injuries, 49–50
reconstruction, 50–52
rehabilitation, 53–56
re-tears, 53
ruptures, 47–48, 50
tears, 2, 49–50
*see also* knee
anti-inflammatories
    bleeding and, 31, 38
    for tendonitis, 66, 85
Apri, Necip, 1
Arlovski, Andrei "The Pit Bull," 12
Arroyo, Matt, 178
arthritis, 63
articular cartilage, 61, 63
Association of Ringside Physicians, 2
axe-kicks, 65

B ——————————————

balance exercises, 71 *fig*
Barnett, Josh
    on educating yourself, 162–163
    on elbow pads, 35–36

on hand injuries, 119
on introspective approach to
    training, 176–177
on live training, 16
on overtraining, 169–170
on shoulder dislocation, 81
on training partners, 161
Baroni, Phil, 56
biceps
    ruptures at elbow, 87–88
    ruptures from shoulder, 86–87
    tendonitis, 86
    tenodesis, 86–87
bleeding
    anti-inflammatories and, 31
    arterial, 28
    compression for, 30
    in the eye, 39
    fight-stopping, 28–30
    venous, 28–29
box jumps, 74 *fig*
boxer's fracture, 118, 126 *fig*
    treatment of, 119–120
boxer's knuckle, 128
boxing gloves
    eye injuries and, 41
    vs MMA gloves, 41, 121, 163–164
    protection of hands, 117, 120, 124
    for sparring, 164
brachialis muscle, 87
brain
    anatomy, 10–11
    baseline testing, 18
brain injury
    chronic brain damage, 21–22
    contrecoup injury, 10
    coup injury, 10
    long-term consequences of, 19–22
    post-concussion syndrome, 12
    second-impact syndrome, 11
    sub-concussive episode, 11
    *see also* concussion; head injury

Brown, Matt "The Immortal," on
    injury prevention, 175–176
Buffer, Bruce, 52
    on concussion, 12
bursitis, 103
butterfly stretches, 106

C ——————————————

cadaver grafts, 51–52
Carter, Shonie, 62
Charuto, 40
chronic brain damage, 21–22
chronic traumatic encephalopathy
    (CTE), 22
clavicle, 80
closed-chain exercises, 78 *fig*
coaches
    choice of, 158–159
    keeping fighters safe, 166–167,
        169–170
    qualities of, 166–167
cold sores, 145–146
Coleman, Mark "The Hammer,"
    39–40
    on ACL tears, 54
    on choice of training partner, 160
    on concussion, 10
    on prevention of hip injury,
        104–105
    on stretching, 160
    on warming up, 92
compression
    enswell for, 27
    lacerations and, 30–31
compression shorts, 101
compression-sleeve braces, 57
concussion, 2
    knockout and, 9–11
    misunderstanding severity of, 9–10
    slurred speech and, 12
    symptoms, 10, 12–13
    *see also* brain injury; head injury

Condit, Carlos, 47–48, 49
　on choice of training
　　environment, 159
　on hand exercises, 124
　on rehabilitation, 55–56
　on sparring, 15–16
　on warming up, 93
confidence, loss of, 120
contrecoup injury, 10
coracoid process, 82 *fig*, 86
core strength exercise, 71 *fig*
Cormier, Daniel, 152
cornea, abrasions of, 38
cortisone, 62–63
　complications from, 85
　for knee injuries, 62–63
　for shoulder injuries, 84–85
　for tendonitis, 66
Côté, Patrick "The Predator," 62
　on ACL tears, 54–55
coup injury, 10
Couture, Randy, 37, 104, 114, 147
　on neck muscle strengthening, 23
　on overtraining, 168–169, 172
　on training environment, 68, 158
cross-training, 172–173
　active rest and, 173–174
Cruz, Dominick, 51
cutman, 27, 28, 31–33
cuts. *see* lacerations

D ———————————————

Danzig, Mac, 31
dashboard injury, 60
Davis, Marcus, 27–28
　on dehydration, 152–153
dehydration, 2, 87–88
　weight-cutting and, 151–152, 153
DellaGrotte, Mark
　on concussion, 11
　on hand injuries, 117
　on hand wrapping, 130–131

on headgear, 164
on injury prevention, 178
on judo throws, 79
on knee injuries, 62–63
on lacerations, 27–28, 31
on padding during training, 33
on skin infections, 147–148
top three injuries, 63
on training smart, 177–178
deltoid muscle, 80
dementia pugilistica, 22
depression, brain injury and, 13, 21–22
Dewees, Edwin, 147
Diaz, Nick, 32, 40, 62, 106
Diaz brothers, 17
diet pills, weight-cutting and, 152
distal interphalangeal (DIP) joint,
　118 *fig*
dos Santos, Junior, 89
drug addiction, 114
Dullanty, Kelly, 87
Duran, Jacob "Stitch," 27, 29–30, 32–33
　on hand wrapping, 130–131
　as teacher, 163
dynamic exercises, 56, 67
dynamic stretching, 106

E ———————————————

eccentric exercises, 111 *fig*
Edgar, Frankie, 170, 171
ego
　grappling and, 68, 168
　training and, 165–166
　in training partners, 159
elbow pads, 35
elbows
　biceps rupture, 87–88
　facial injuries from, 35, 37, 40
electrolyte imbalances, weight-cutting
　and, 152
enswell, 27, 30–31
epinephrine for lacerations, 31, 32–33

equipment
proper use of, 41, 163–165
sanitizing of, 147–148, 149
escape techniques, 69
Estwanik, Joe, on ringside medicine,
1–4
Evans, Rashad, 92
exercises
balance, 71 *fig*
chest press, 99 *fig*
closed-chain, 78 *fig*
core strength, 71 *fig*
dynamic, 56, 67
eccentric, 111 *fig*
hand injury prevention, 121–123,
124
hip strength and flexibility, 108
*fig*–112 *fig*
knee injury prevention, 71 *fig*–78 *fig*
lunge, 58, 72 *fig*–73 *fig*, 109 *fig*
neck muscle strengthening, 22–23,
24 *fig*–26 *fig*
newspaper ball exercise, 122 *fig*–123
*fig*
open-chain, 78 *fig*
pelvic lifts, 112 *fig*
plank exercises, 110 *fig*
plyometrics, 56, 67, 74 *fig*
resistance bands, 74 *fig*, 95 *fig*
reverse curls, 99 *fig*
rotator cuff, 96 *fig*
rowing, 100 *fig*
shoulder injury prevention, 94
*fig*–100 *fig*
stretching, 98 *fig*
warming up, 95 *fig*, 99 *fig*
extensor tendons, 118 *fig*, 127–128
eye injuries
abrasions, 38
blunt trauma, 38–39
boxing gloves and, 41
MMA gloves and, 41
retinal damage, 38–39

rupture of globe, 39
treatment of, 38
eye pokes, 41
eye protection, 40–41

F ————————————————

face
lacerations, 27
zones of concern for laceration,
35 *fig*
facial injuries, 37–38
falls, proper technique for, 106–107
fasting, weight-cutting and, 152
femur, 48, 50 *fig*, 101, 102 *fig*
FightMedicine.net, 6
Filipovic, Mirko "Cro Cop," 81
finger dislocations, 124–126
MMA gloves and, 124–125
flexibility
exercises for, 106
hip exercises, 108 *fig*–112 *fig*
importance of, 59, 176
flexor tendons, 118 *fig*, 127–128
flexor digitorum profundis
tendon, 118 *fig*
flexor digitorum superficialis
tendon, 118 *fig*
floaters (eye), 38–39
Florian, Kenny, 84
flow in training, 159
foam rollers, 106, 109 *fig*
follicle-stimulating hormone (FSH), 154
Foster, Andy
on choice of training partner, 64–65
on hand wrapping, 131
on knee injuries, 64–65
on mouthguards, 164–165
on sparring, 16
frontal lobe dysfunction, 21–22
Frye, Don "The Predator," 18
on choice of training partner, 160
on hand injuries, 124
on lacerations, 34

on orbital fractures, 39
on stretching, 160
on Vaseline, 34
functional training, 176
fungal infections, 148–149

G

Gamburyan, Manny, 114
gamekeeper's thumb, 125
gi (uniform), 123–124, 149
glenoid, 80, 82 *fig*
gloves
    boxing gloves, 41, 121, 163–164
    hand protection and, 117, 120, 124
    MMA gloves, 16, 17, 41, 121, 124–
        125, 163–164
Gomi, Takanori, 40
gonadotropin-releasing hormone
    (GnRH), 154
governing body, need for, 153
Gracie, Cesar, 32
    on cortisone, 66
    on eye injuries, 40–41
    on hand injuries, 120
    on headgear, 34
    on hip injuries, 106
    on resistance bands, 92–93
    on shoulder injuries, 91
    on sparring, 17
    on tendonitis, 66
    on Vaseline, 34
    on yoga, 174
Gracie, Renzo
    on choice of training partner, 162
    on concussion, 13
    on good coaches, 167
    on head injury during training, 14
    on overtraining, 170
    on resistance bands, 92
    on taking time to heal, 128
Gracie, Royce, 5
Gracie Jiu-Jitsu, 5
grappling

with a gi, 123–124
knee injuries, 64–65, 69
ligament tears and, 49, 58
mats, 68
MMA gloves for, 41, 163–164
neuromuscular control, 67
stretching before, 115
visualization and, 44
grappling gloves. *see* MMA gloves
gravity boots, 176
greater trochanter, 102 *fig*
    snapping hips and, 103
grip strength, 121–123, 122 *fig*–123 *fig*
groin pulls, 103

H

Hackleman, John, 89
Hall, Mark, 39
hamstrings, 102
    grafts, 51
    ruptures, 104
    tears, 113–115
hand, anatomy of, 117–118, 118 *fig*
hand exercises, 121–123
hand injuries, 117–118
    boxer's fracture, 118, 126 *fig*
    finger dislocations, 124–126
    fractures, 118–120
    prevention of, 121–124
    tendon injuries, 126–128, 127 *fig*
    treatment of, 119–120
hand wrapping, 120, 121, 130–131, 164
    techniques, 132 *fig*–144 *fig*
head injury
    pituitary dysfunction after, 155
    prevention of, 14–15
    symptoms, 21–22
    during training, 14
    *see also* brain injury; concussion
head-butts, 34
headgear
    injury prevention and, 34
    during training, 14–15, 40, 163, 164

heel hooks, knee injuries and, 69

Henderson, Benson, 79, 171

Henderson, Matt, 13

Herman, Ed, 49, 51–52

    on ACL tears, 53–54, 55

herpes, 145–146

herpes gladiatorum, 146

hip

    anatomy of, 101–102, 102 *fig*

    bursitis, 103

    snapping hips, 103–104

hip exercises, 108 *fig*–112 *fig*

hip flexors, 102–103, 106

hip injuries, 101–104

    adductor injuries, 102–103

    judo throws and, 106

    prevention of, 104–107

hip replacements, 104–105

Hodge, Danny, 123

Holm, Holly, 15

Hughes, Matt, 13, 113–114, 164

Hume, Matt, 166

humerus, 80

Hunt, Mark, on PCL injuries, 61

hyphema, 38

hypogonadism, 155

I ———————————————

ice

    for hand injuries, 124, 131

    as recovery tool, 174

iliac crest, 102 *fig*

iliopsoas tendon, 102 *fig*

    snapping hips and, 103

iliotibial (IT) band, 102 *fig*

    stretches, 108 *fig*

impetigo, 146–148

infections, prevention of, 32–33

infraorbital nerve, 29

infraspinatus, 80 *fig*, 83

injuries

    increase in incidence of, 6

    working around, 167–168

injury prevention, 39

    avoidance of overtraining, 168–172

    lack of resources for, 6–7

    listening to your body, 165–166

    mental preparation and, 43–45

    principles of, 7, 157

    in training camp, 14, 178

    *see also specific injuries, e.g. shoulder injuries*

insurance, 6, 179

J ———————————————

Jackson, Greg, 35, 55–56, 67

Jackson, Quinton "Rampage," 113

jersey finger, 128

Jiu-Jitsu, 5, 68

    grip strength and, 123

    hand injuries and, 123–124

    hip injuries, 105

    meniscus injuries, 62

Johnson, Demetrious

    on hand injuries, 119–120

    on insurance, 179

    on labral tears, 89–90

    on listening to your body, 165–166

    on skin infections, 146

    on training, 182

Johnston, Brian, 39, 124

Jones, Jon, 15, 35, 37, 67, 89, 92

judo

    hip injuries and, 106

    knee injuries and, 56, 68

    shoulder injuries and, 79

    throws, 79

K ———————————————

Kennedy, Tim

    on ACL tears, 55

    on injury prevention, 70

    on mental stimulation, 173–174

    on quadriceps tendon injuries, 65–66

Klitschko brothers, 32

knee
    anatomy of, 48, 50 *fig*
    braces, 57
    ligaments, 48, 50 *fig*
    menisci, 48, 50 *fig*
    *see also* anterior cruciate ligament
        (ACL)
knee bars, 69
knee exercises, 71 *fig*–78 *fig*
knee injuries
    ACL injuries, 49–58
    causes of, 69
    LCL injuries, 60
    MCL injuries, 58–60
    meniscus injuries, 61–65
    patellar tendon injuries, 65–66
    PCL injuries, 60–61
    prevention of, 59, 64–65, 67–70
    quadriceps tendon injuries, 65–66
knockouts
    concussion and, 9–13
    preventing, 22
    in training camp, 15
Kondo, Yuki, 9

L ————————————

labral tears, 88–90
labrum
    hip, 101, 102 *fig*
    shoulder, 80, 82 *fig*
    tears, 88–90, 101, 103
lacerations
    compression and, 30–31
    fight-stopping, 29–30
    healing time for, 32
    hygiene and, 33
    long-term consequences of, 28
    nerve damage and, 29
    prevention of, 33–36
    suturing, 32
    treatment for, 30–32
    Vaseline and, 31, 33
    zones of concern, 35 *fig*

Laimon, Marc, 147
"last week curse," 168
lateral collateral ligament (LCL), 48,
    50 *fig*
    injuries, 60
latissimus dorsi, 80, 100 *fig*
Lauzon, Joe, 31
Lawler, Robbie, 164, 166
laxatives, weight-cutting and, 152
Le Banner, Jérôme, 61
leg locks, knee injuries and, 69–70
Lesnar, Brock, 69, 89, 167
Lewis, John, 166
Liborio, Ricardo
    on grappling with a gi, 123–124
    on hip injuries, 105
    on labral tears, 89
    on training environment, 68
Lindland, Matt, on great teammates,
    161–162
Lister, Dean
    on choice of training partner, 64
    on concussion, 13–14
    on knee injuries, 64
    on lacerations, 33
    on "last week curse," 168
    on shoulder injuries, 91
    on skin infections, 148
live training, 16, 69, 181–182
long extensor tendon, 118 *fig*
Longo, Ray
    on biceps rupture, 87–88
    on hand injuries, 129
    on keeping fighters safe, 172
    on meniscus injuries, 62
losing your chin, 17
Ludwig, Duane "Bang," 64
lunge exercises, 58, 72 *fig*–73 *fig*, 109 *fig*
luteinizing hormone (LH), 154
Lytle, Chris, 34, 62

M ————————————

Machida, Lyoto, 129

mallet finger, 127
Markham, Rory, 153
mats
   choice of, 68, 106–107, 163
   sanitizing of, 147, 149
McCarthy, "Big John," 2
   on concussion, 20–21
medial collateral ligament (MCL), 48,
   50 *fig*
   injuries, 58–60
meditation, 44–45
Melendez, Gilbert, 17
   on AC separations, 83
   on concussion, 11
   on MCL injuries, 59–60
   on overtraining, 171
   on prevention of hip injury, 106
   on protective gear, 164
   on shoulder injuries, 91
   on taping hands, 126
Melendez, Gilbert Sr., on shoulder
   injuries, 79
Mendez, Javier
   on labral tears, 89–90
   on sparring, 17
menisci
   injuries, 61–65
   repair of, 63–64
   shaving of, 63
mental preparation, 43–45
mental stimulation, 173–174
metacarpal bones, 118 *fig*
   fractures of, 118–119
metacarpophalangeal (MCP) joint, 118
   *fig*, 118–119
Methicillin-resistant Staphylococcus
   aureus (MRSA), 146–147
Mezger, Guy, on brain health, 18–19
Miletich, Pat
   on choice of gloves, 164
   on cross-training, 172
   on functional training, 176
   on gravity boots, 176

on MCL injuries, 59
on MMA gloves, 41
on neck injury, 23
on newspaper ball exercise, 123
on padding during training, 164
on rotator cuff injuries, 83–84
on safer training and fighting, 39,
   166–167
on training, 182
on working around injuries,
   167–168
Miller, Jason "Mayhem," 113
Miocic, Stipe, 24
MMA gloves
   vs boxing gloves, 41, 121, 163–164
   eye injuries and, 41
   finger dislocations and, 124–125
   proper use of, 163, 164
   in training, 16, 17, 41
Monson, Jeff
   on active rest, 173
   on warming up, 176
mouthguards, 164–165
MRSA, 146–147
Muay Thai, 5, 59–60
   choice of training partner in, 65
muscular stability
   drills for, 59
   importance of, 56

N ————————————

nasolacrimal duct, 29
neck strengthening, 19, 22–23
   exercises, 24 *fig*–26 *fig*
Nelson, Greg
   on AC separations, 84
   on good coaches, 167
   on injury prevention, 175
   on knee injuries, 69–70
   on rotator cuff injuries, 84–85
   on training camps, 180–182
nerve damage, lacerations and, 29
newspaper ball exercise, 122 *fig*–123 *fig*

Newton, Carlos
    on biceps tenodesis, 86–87
    on injury prevention, 68–69
    on learning how to fall, 106–107
    on orbital fractures, 40
    on overtraining, 171–172
    on prevention of hand injuries, 121
Nogueira, Antônio Rodrigo
    "Minotauro," 104

O ———————————

open-chain exercises, 78 *fig*
optic nerve, injuries to, 38
orbital fractures, 37, 39–40
Ortiz, Tito, 58, 113, 121
overtraining
    avoiding, 168–172
    signs of, 170, 172, 173
Owen, Steve, 39

P ———————————

painkillers, addiction to, 114
Parisyan, Karo, 62
    on hamstring injuries, 113–115
    on warming up, 115
patella, 48, 50 *fig*
patellar tendon, 50 *fig*, 51
    grafts, 50–51
    inflammation of, 66
    injuries, 65–66
patellar tendonitis, 66
pelvic lifts, 112 *fig*
Penn, BJ, 30, 101
performance enhancing drugs (PEDs),
    154–156
Perretti, John, 2
personality changes, brain injury and,
    21–22
phalangeal bones, 118
physical therapy, 55, 103
pituitary dysfunction, 155
plank exercises, 110 *fig*
platelet-rich plasma (PRP), 66–67, 89

plyometrics, 56, 62, 67, 74 *fig*
post-concussion syndrome, 12
posterior cruciate ligament (PCL), 48,
    50 *fig*
    injuries, 60–61
prehab, 52, 175
proximal interphalangeal (PIP) joint,
    118 *fig*, 118–119
Pulver, Jens, 164, 166
punch-drunk syndrome, 22
punching
    hand wrapping and, 164
    safe methods for, 118, 121, 130

Q ———————————

quadriceps, 102
quadriceps tendon, 50 *fig*
    injuries, 65–66
Quarry, Nate "Rock"
    on choice of training partner,
        159–160
    on overtraining, 169
    on training smart, 179

R ———————————

record keeping, 171–172
rehabilitation
    after ACL tear, 53–56
    after labral tear, 89–90
    after rotator cuff injury, 85
    after SLAP tear, 90–91
resistance bands
    exercises, 74 *fig*, 95 *fig*
    for shoulder injuries, 91, 92–93
rest
    importance of, 128, 171
    scheduling, 169–170, 181
    *see also* active rest
retina, injuries to, 38
ringside medicine, 1–4
ringworm, 148–149
rotator cuff, 80–81
    surgery, 84

tears, 83–85
tendonitis, 83–85
rotator cuff exercises, 96 *fig*
running drills, 77 *fig*
Rutten, Bas "El Guapo"
    on biceps tendonitis, 86
    on overtraining, 171
    on protective gear, 164

## S

Sauer, Pedro, 70
scapula, 82 *fig*
scar tissue, 27–28
    build up of, 32, 114
Schaub, Brendan, 104
second-impact syndrome, 11
Serra, Matt, 147–148, 172
    on biceps rupture, 87–88
    on changing training habits,
        178–179
    on headgear, 34
    on meniscus injuries, 62
Severn, Dan, 5
    on cross-training, 172–173
    on good training camps, 162
    on injury prevention, 175
    on sanitizing of equipment, 149
    on skin infections, 148–149
shadowboxing, 45
Shamrock, Frank, 57
    on ACL tears, 56–57
    on brain injuries, 9–10
    on ice as recovery tool, 174
    on injury prevention, 44
    on mental preparation, 43–45
    on neck muscle strengthening, 22
    on padding during training, 163
    on prevention of hand injuries, 121
    on sanitizing of equipment, 149
    on SLAP lesion, 90–91
Shamrock, Ken, 5
    on ACL tears, 57–58
    finger dislocation, 125 *fig*

on hand injuries, 125
on hip injuries, 105–106
on meniscus injuries, 64
neck injury, 21 *fig*, 22–23
on prevention of hand injuries,
    121–123
Sherk, Sean "The Muscle Shark," 69,
    167
    on functional training, 176
    on hand wrapping and ice, 131
    on hip injuries, 101
    on injury prevention, 70
    on lacerations, 33–34
    shoulder injuries, 84–85
    on skin infections, 148
Shields, Jake, 11, 17, 52, 79
shoulder, anatomy of, 80 *fig*, 80–81,
    82 *fig*
shoulder injuries
    AC separations, 82–83
    dislocation, 81–82
    judo throws and, 79
    prevention of, 90–91
    rehabilitation, 90–93
    rotator cuff, 83–85
    shaking bow for, 90
Silva, Anderson, 62–63
Silva, Antonio "Bigfoot," 61
Silva, Thiago, 37
Simpson, Aaron, 49
Sinosic, Elvis, 90
skier's thumb, 125
skin infections
    herpes, 145–146
    impetigo, 146–148
    ringworm, 148–149
    staphylococcus, 32, 146–148
    streptococcus, 146
SLAP lesions, 88–91
    treatment for, 88–90
slow physical forms, 45, 91
slurred speech, 12
snapping hips, 103–104

sparring
    after head injury, 14
    after lacerations, 32
    drills, 182
    equipment for, 164
    gloves for, 120
    hand wrapping for, 131
    with heavier opponents, 17–18
    limiting, 3, 11, 15–17, 19
Sperry, Mario, on hand injuries,
    130–131
sports medicine, MMA and, 2, 7
Spratt, Pete
    on ruptured thumb tendon, 128
    ruptured thumb tendon, 127 *fig*
standard of care, 2
staphylococcus infections, 32, 146–148
starvation, 2
    weight-cutting and, 152
Stevenson, Joe, 30
"Stitch." *see* Duran, Jacob "Stitch"
St-Pierre, Georges, 34, 52, 55–56, 62,
    147, 162
    hip injury, 102–103
    knee injury, 47–48, 53
    knee reconstruction, 50–51
strength and conditioning, 177, 181
streptococcus, 146
stretching
    hip, 108 *fig*–109 *fig*
    importance of, 23, 160, 181
    shoulder, 90, 92, 98 *fig*
striking
    gloves for, 41, 163–164
    hand injuries and, 117–119, 121
Struve, Stefan, 61
sub-concussive injuries, 3, 11
subscapularis, 80 *fig*, 83
supplements, 156
supraorbital nerve, 29, 35 *fig*
supraspinatus, 80 *fig*, 83
Sylvia, Tim, 164, 166
    on active rest, 174

on concussion, 12
on confidence, 120
synthetic testosterone, 154

T ——————————————

t'ai chi, 45
takedowns, 166–167
    vs judo throws, 79
    knee injuries and, 65
Taktarov, Oleg, 128
Teixeira, Glover, 89
Telligman, Tra, 57
tendonitis
    biceps, 86
    exercises for, 111 *fig*
    patellar tendon, 66
    rotator cuff, 83–85
    treatment for, 66, 85
tensor fasciae latae, 102 *fig*
teres minor, 83
testosterone
    synthetic, 154
    weight-cutting and, 155
testosterone replacement therapy
    (TRT), 154–155
Thompson, Nick, 114
tibia, 48, 50 *fig*
tinea corporis, 148–149
training
    changing habits in, 178–179
    functional approach to, 176
    introspective approach to, 176–177
    training smarter vs training harder,
        175–179
training camps
    choice of, 159–160, 162
    extending, 171
    individualizing, 172
    injury prevention in, 178
    planning, 180–182
training environment
    choice of, 67–68, 106
    continuity in, 158

training partners
    choice of, 34, 64–65, 158–159, 160
    ego in, 159
    qualities of, 161–162
trapezius, 81, 100 *fig*
traumatic brain injury. *see* brain injury
Trigg, Frank, 23

V ───────────────

Vaseline, 163, 164
    lacerations and, 31, 33, 34
Velasquez, Cain, 89–90, 171
Vera, Brandon
    on choice of training partner,
        158–159
    on facial injuries, 37–38
    on injury prevention, 174
visualization, 43–44
Vovchanchyn, Igor, 57

W───────────────

warming up, 182
    exercises, 95 *fig*, 99 *fig*
    importance of, 115, 176
    knees, 59
    shoulders, 90–93
water resistance training, 83–84
Weidman, Chris, 128–129, 172

weight-cutting
    dehydration and, 151–152
    diet pills and, 152
    effect on testosterone levels, 155
    electrolyte imbalances and, 152
    health issues around, 151–154
    laxatives and, 152
    safe levels for, 153–154
White, Dana, 114, 147
Williams, Pete, 10, 54
Winkeljohn, Mike, 35
    on eye injuries, 41
    on hand wrapping, 131
    on neck muscle strengthening, 22
    on prevention of head injury, 14–15
    on stretching, 92
    on training environment, 67–68
Woodley, Tyron, 49
wrapping of hands. *see* hand wrapping
wrestling
    hip injuries and, 105–106
    skin infections and, 146

Y ───────────────

yoga, 45, 160, 174

Z ───────────────

Zingano, Cat, 51